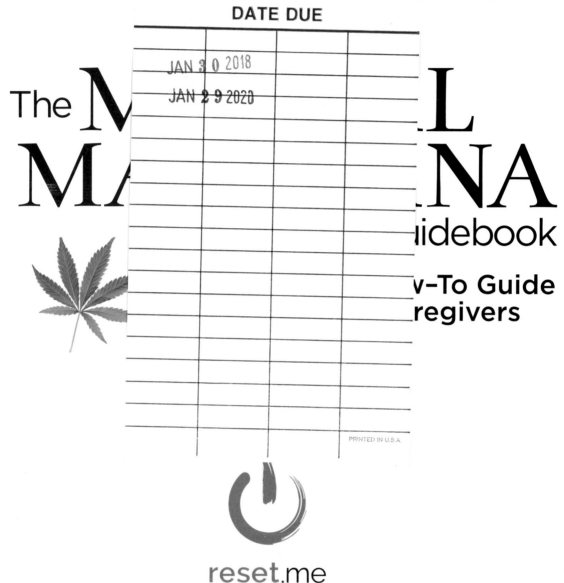

The M____ MA____ ____L ____NA idebook

v-To Guide regivers

reset.me

David Downs

**This book is dedicated to my father,
Robert James Downs**

The Medical Marijuana Guidebook

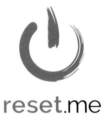

reset.me

© 2016 Reset.me
3101 Clairmont Road • Suite G • Atlanta, GA 30329

Correspondence concerning this book may be directed to Reset.me, Attn: *The Medical Marijuana Guidebook*, at the address above.

ISBN: 0794843727
Printed in the United States of America

Please visit our website at Reset.me.

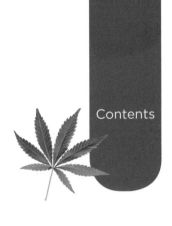

Contents

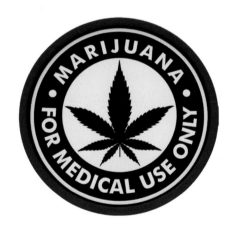

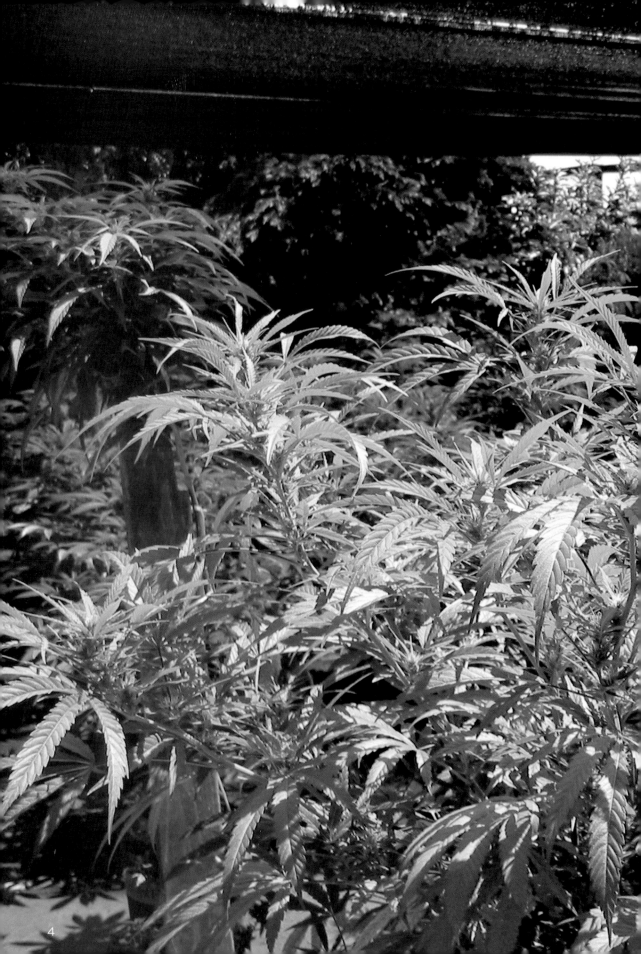

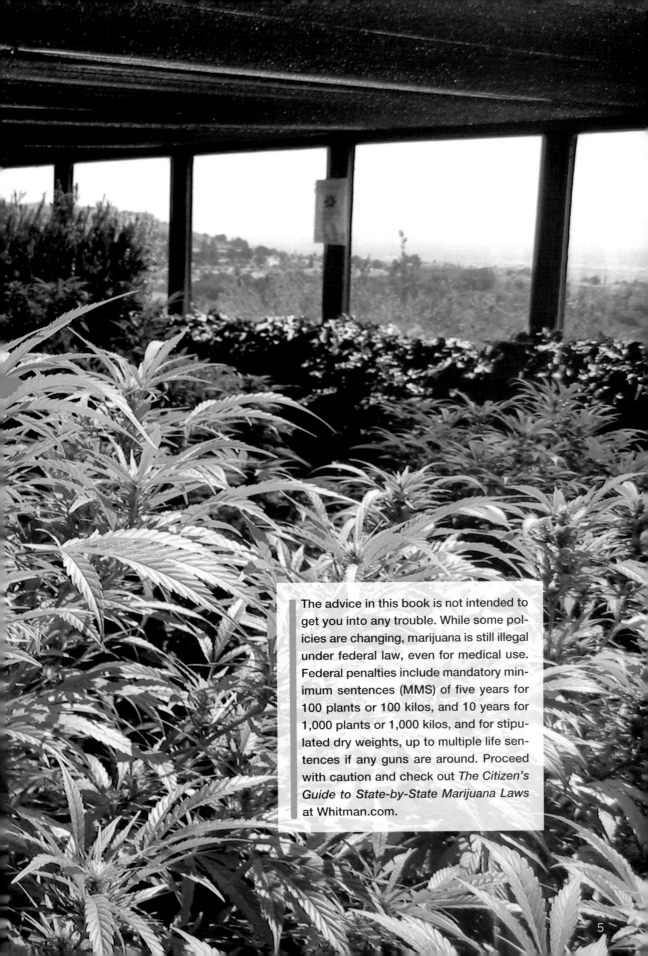

The advice in this book is not intended to get you into any trouble. While some policies are changing, marijuana is still illegal under federal law, even for medical use. Federal penalties include mandatory minimum sentences (MMS) of five years for 100 plants or 100 kilos, and 10 years for 1,000 plants or 1,000 kilos, and for stipulated dry weights, up to multiple life sentences if any guns are around. Proceed with caution and check out *The Citizen's Guide to State-by-State Marijuana Laws* at Whitman.com.

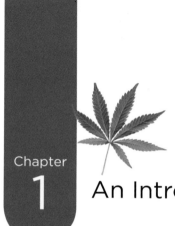

An Introduction To Medical Marijuana

"My partner has cancer. My doctor said we're running out of options and recommended medical marijuana. But that's all he would say. What do we do?"

Many people have asked this question. Since 2009, I've written the award-winning, syndicated column "Legalization Nation" for the *East Bay Express* in Oakland, California, and other newspapers. Appearing in print weekly or bi-weekly, along with daily web postings, the column has hit a nerve.

People have many great, valid questions about medical marijuana. This book answers their most frequent questions succinctly and accurately, backed up by citations of the most current, acceptable, and primary sources of medical science and law.

This book exists because patients have directly asked me for it, and you can't ignore someone facing cancer, or who has a loved one with a serious disease.

This guidebook is the world's first book to pair concise, accurate, practical information about medical cannabis usage with the current law. Many books can tell you about cannabis' history, or about strains, or how to grow it. The medical science is widely available to anyone with an Internet connection. Several databases also attempt to track medical marijuana laws on a state-by-state basis.

But this book puts the law and the practical application of it together the same way patients across America have to do every single day.

We distilled this book into four main parts: the Basics, the Details, a State-By-State Guide, and Resources for further assistance.

In the Basics, you'll find the most essential overview needed to begin accessing medical cannabis in the United States.

> "Cannabis has been a medicine for a lot longer than it hasn't been."
>
> – *Dr. Donald Abrams, M.D.*

In the Details, we explore the types of cannabis products, the plant's active ingredients, dosage, and how patients use different formulations of cannabis.

In our State-By-State Guide, we explain the unique steps you take in each state to access medical cannabis, and how they can vary widely.

And finally, in our Resources section, you can find ways to continue getting help accessing medical cannabis, including further details on how to find a doctor that recommends cannabis, how to find caregivers, dispensa-

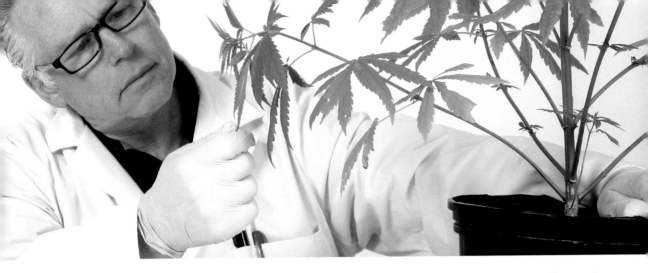

ries and other outlets, advice for prospective homegrowers, and advice for medical cannabis refugees who are leaving their home state to obtain the medicine.

There's no way we can cover every use case and scenario in this book, so we're trying to cover the most common ones, and if you have any further questions, you can contact us through our website at www.usmmj.org and we'll do our best to help.

If the column that inspired this book has had any success, it's because it was conceived with one primary goal: to be of service to its readers. We hope this book will be of service to you or someone you love, as well.

How to Legally Obtain Medical Marijuana in the U.S.

While there is an incredible variance in what people can get medical cannabis for, and how they can get it, there are some national commonalities. Everywhere medical cannabis is legal in the U.S., you have to have a qualifying medical condition, get a doctor's recommendation for cannabis, perhaps enroll in a state program, then find and obtain the drug in the appropriate form, use it safely, and determine if the formulation is effective or should be adjusted.

Indication

All legal medical marijuana use starts with a qualifying disease or symptom like cancer or chronic pain. Every state has a different list of such diseases or symptoms that allows a patient to qualify for the state's law. These indications normally include diseases or symptoms like chronic pain, chronic muscle spasms, cancer, HIV and AIDS, or wasting. There are dozens of indications for medical cannabis use — from business professionals managing chronic anxiety, to hospice patients easing the pain, nausea and depression of a terminal illness, to kids with catastrophic epilepsy.

Recommendation

No matter what medical cannabis state you live in, to be a legal patient, you're going to need to find a doctor to write, sign and date a recommendation for

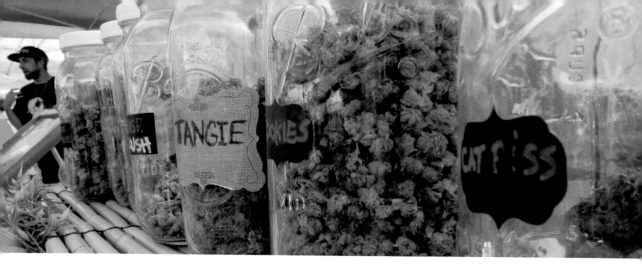

you to use cannabis medicinally. These recommendations can be cheap and easy to obtain in places like California and Oregon, or they can be impossible to get, as in many states in the South.

Sometimes it's your primary care physician who recommends cannabis after all treatments have failed. However, most doctors are not yet taught about cannabis medicines in medical school[1]. So most often, a patient seeks out a specialist physician who is experienced in determining if a patient might benefit from using the botanical. Sometimes doctors can simply hand-write a recommendation, but many states require doctors to fill out a specific form online, and others add more layers of red tape.

State Program

While all legal patients must have a doctor's recommendation, participating in a state program is also sometimes mandatory. These state programs primarily consist of official registries where patients sign up to get an identification card. States often use these confidential registries to verify valid patients during police stops and other law enforcement activity. In many states, registration is mandatory to enjoy the legal protections of a medical marijuana law.

Signing up for a state's program can be as simple as downloading, printing out and signing a one-page form, or it can be very, very lengthy and expensive, with multiple forms to fill out, fingerprinting, background checks, and steep annual fees of up to $200 per patient.

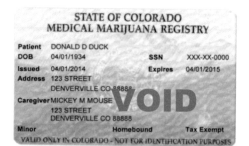

Acquisition

After you get a doctor's recommendation, and sign up for your mandatory state registration (if required), you're going to need to find a way to acquire the medicine.

Obtaining medical cannabis legally in the United States can be very easy in places like California, where delivery services will bring it to your door with the push of a button on your smartphone, or it can be next to impossible in parts of the Midwest, South and Eastern United States.

States with the best access to medical cannabis will have retail stores (dispensaries) that sell the drug the same way you buy any other retail item. Some states allow private groups (collectives or cooperatives) to grow and share marijuana.

Other patients chose to grow cannabis themselves or have a caregiver do it, if legally permitted under state medical marijuana law.

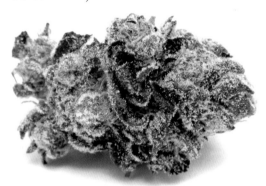

Many Midwest, Eastern and Southern states have medical marijuana laws, but no legal way to obtain the drug in the state. The United States also has a thriving illicit market in cannabis in nearly every city and town.

Type

By far the most commonly available form of medical cannabis in the state is raw, dried cannabis plants — specifically, the unfertilized female flower buds of the plant, which are the most medically active.

Where medical cannabis is more legal, there are more processed formulations available, including:

— medically infused foods and other products (edibles).

— potent extracts of cannabis (hash, oil, tincture, etc.).

— topical products for use externally on the skin.

Medically infused foods and other products (edibles).

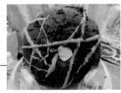

The first pharmaceutical industry formulations of cannabis extract — Sativex™ and Epidiolex™ from GW Pharmaceuticals — are just becoming available on a very limited basis in the United States.

Use

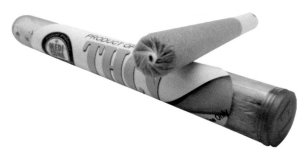

Smoked: The most common way people use cannabis medicinally is also one of the simplest and cheapest: they smoke it. Raw, dried, female flower buds are chopped or ground and placed in a pipe or rolled into a paper, exposed to open flame, burned and the resulting smoke is inhaled. The open flame releases the plant's active ingredients, which are inhaled and cross into the body via the lungs. Smoking causes effects that begin in less than a minute, and it allows patients to easily adjust dosing.

Eaten: One of the most inviting ways for medical patients who do not want to smoke is infused foods and products, called edibles. The producer infuses the active ingredients in cannabis into an oil or other carrying substance that is then baked into a food or added to a drink. The plant's active ingredients are swallowed and enter the body through the stomach. Eating edibles causes slower-acting but more intense effects than smoking, and dosing is more difficult.

Vaporized: Patients who want to avoid smoke but want fast-acting effects have begun using vaporizers,

which can be as large as a toaster or as small as a ballpoint pen. Vaporizers use far lower temperatures than burning to create medically active vapor without the irritants of burning plants. Vaporizers work with flowers and/or extracts, and dosing can be either very precise or very difficult depending on formulation and modality

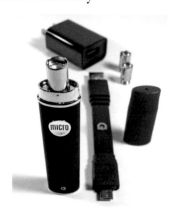

Extracts: Patients are also rapidly adopting the use of extracts of cannabis in legal medical marijuana states. These extracts are similar to the essential oils of any other plant, and they can be oil-like, waxy or granular. Extracts are multiple times more potent than raw plants. Dosing can be difficult — or easier — depending on modality. When combined with portable micro-vaporizers (vape pens), extracts can be used virtually anywhere without drawing unwanted attention.

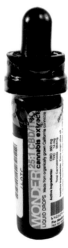

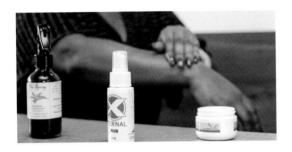

Topicals: Patients are applying to their skin special balms, lotions and creams that are infused with the active ingredients of cannabis. These topicals have been reported to treat a wide variety of intractable skin conditions like eczema and psoriasis, and they're also used like muscle ointment to calm nerve and muscle inflammation, pain and tension. Dosing is generally not an issue with topicals.

Adjust or Discontinue

As patients begin acquiring and using medical cannabis, they begin to hone in on the right source of cannabis, the right type of cannabis, their preferred formulation of it, and a mode of delivery that best suits their condition and situation. The process is similar to trying an over-the-counter drug. Doctor recommendations are usually good for one year (though some are as good for as little as 30 days), and your doctor may ask you how cannabis is working for you, and recommend adjustments to type, formulation and mode of use. If the medical condition has resolved, you may be asked to discontinue use.

Applicable States

The state of medical marijuana laws is changing almost every week. At press time, medical marijuana laws exist in 23 states, 16 states have a law related to the cannabis ingredient cannabidiol (CBD) on their books, and 11 states have no medical cannabis law whatsoever.

You generally have to be a resident of a state to enjoy its medical marijuana laws. Residency is often proven by submitting a copy of recent utility bill or copy of valid driver's license or state identification card. Patients who are traveling to another state to receive medical care, or moving to another state to access medical cannabis, may have to obtain one of these documents to begin using a program.

> "[T]he risk of marijuana use in states before passing medical marijuana laws did not differ significantly from the risk after medical marijuana laws were passed. Results were generally robust across sensitivity analyses, including redefining marijuana use as any use in the previous year or frequency of use, and re-analysing medical marijuana laws for delayed effects or for variation in provisions for dispensaries."
>
> — "Medical marijuana laws and adolescent marijuana use in the USA from 1991 to 2014: results from annual, repeated cross-sectional surveys," *Lancet Psychiatry* 2015: 2:601-08

Generally, most states do not recognize each other's medical marijuana laws, but that is changing. Recognizing

STATE MARIJUANA LAWS

Decriminalization · Hemp · Legalization · Medical · Medical CBD

NORML

another state's medical marijuana law is called "reciprocity" and it varies on a state-by-state basis. For example, Nevada recognizes out-of-state patients who have a condition that would qualify under Nevada medical marijuana law.

The applicable medical marijuana states in the U.S. are: Alaska, Arizona, California, Colorado, Connecticut, Delaware, Maine, Maryland, Massachusetts, Michigan, Minnesota, Montana, Nevada, New Hampshire, New Jersey, New Mexico, New York, Oregon, Rhode Island, Vermont and Washington.

The states with a medical CBD law on the books are: Alabama, Florida, Georgia, Illinois, Iowa, Kentucky, Louisiana, Mississippi, Missouri, North Carolina, Oklahoma, South Carolina, Tennessee, Texas, Utah, Virginia, Wisconsin and Wyoming.

States with no medical cannabis law whatsoever are: Arkansas, Idaho, Indiana, Kansas, Nebraska, North Dakota, Ohio, Pennsylvania, South Dakota and West Virginia.

Additionally, four states — Colorado, Washington, Oregon and Alaska — have legalized marijuana for any use

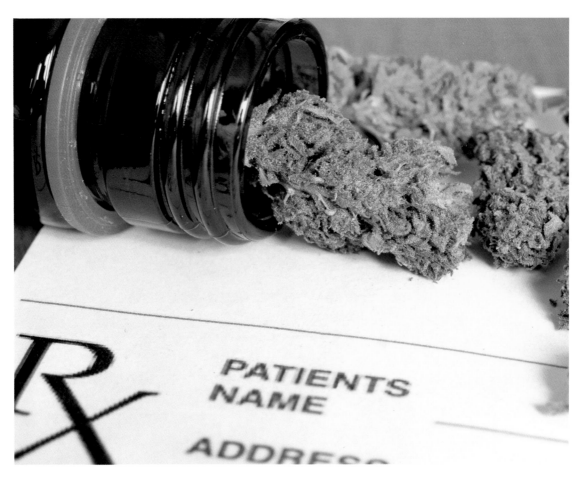

by adults ages 21 and over. Adults can generally possess one ounce of dried bud, grow a few plants, and go to legal retail stores. Recreational legalization provides a greater amount of access and protection to medical cannabis than any medical law. Washington, D.C., also has medical and recreational marijuana legalization, but Congress is blocking cannabis' regulated, commercial distribution.

Just because a state has a medical marijuana law or a CBD law on the books does not mean patients there have legal access to cannabis or any of its formulations. Legal medical marijuana access is very easy in a place like California, but virtually impossible in Wyoming — yet both have medical marijuana laws.

Lastly, most CBD laws are not serving the overwhelmingly vast majority of patients. If you live in a state with a CBD law, chances are, almost no one is getting legal medical cannabis products. (See the State-By-State Guide for ratings on difficulty of legal access, details, and what you can do).

Top Indications for Cannabis Use

Patients are using cannabis for dozens of different diseases and symptoms, but some indications are more popular than others, as measured by patient self-reporting[2][3], qualifying conditions in each state, and state-level registry reporting systems.[4]

Some of the most common indications for medical cannabis use are: severe and chronic pain[5] (including headache and migraines[6]), muscle spasms, seizures, anxiety, arthritis, nausea/appetite/wasting, Crohn's disease, cancer, hepatitis C, glaucoma, and HIV/AIDS.

Like any other drug, cannabis may not treat every indication for which it is listed, for every possible patient in the world, every time it is used.

Count of Patients by Condition and Percentage of Patients Reporting the Condition

Condition	Count of Reporting Patients[2]	Percentage of Reporting Patients
Severe Pain	67,312	92.8%
Spasms	19,886	27.4%
Nausea	9,824	13.5%
Cancer	3,964	5.5%
Seizures	1,948	2.7%
Cachexia	1,168	1.6%
HIV/AIDS	730	1.0%
Glaucoma	1,094	1.5%
Agitation related to Alzheimer's disease	84	.1%
PTSD	4,620	6.4%

Severe and chronic pain

Consistently one of the most common[7] reasons for using medical cannabis is severe, chronic pain — particularly pain associated with nerve damage, called neuropathy[8].[9] Cell and animal studies as well as high-quality[10] clinical trials[11] on humans[12] [13] and patient self-reports consistently conclude[14] [15] that cannabis' active ingredients mediate the pain perception system[16] in humans, and can cause relief.[17][18][19] States with medical marijuana laws have 25 percent less opioid painkiller over-

> "Topicals are very economical and effective for pain from arthritis, injuries, migraines, etc. Since they do not enter the blood stream, they do not cause unwanted psychological effects."
> — *Danielle Schumacher*

doses[20], presumably because cannabis can be a safer[21], less addictive substitute than Vicodin or Oxycontin, and allows chronic pain suffers to consume fewer pills, or quit pills entirely.

Muscle spasms

The active ingredients in cannabis have been shown in cell and animal studies as well as human clinical trials[22] [23] [24] [25]and in patient self-reports to ease chronic, untreatable muscle spasms[26]. These spasms can result from a variety of sources, most commonly including multiple sclerosis[27], and spinal cord injury resulting in paralysis.[28]

Seizures

The active ingredients in cannabis have been shown in cell and animal studies[29] [30]as well as small human studies[31] and in patient self-reports[32] [33] [34] [35]to ease the chronic, severe, incurable seizures that are often associated with epilepsy[36] [37] and traumatic brain injury. Cell and animal studies as well as human clinical trials[38] have shown the active ingredients in cannabis calm overactive nerve activity[39] that can trigger such seizures.

Anxiety

A common and controversial indication for cannabis use is chronic, severe anxiety. Cannabis' active ingredients have been proven in cell and animal studies as well as in human trials[40][41] and patient self-reports[42] to cause sedation[43], which can lead to reduced anxiety among certain patients. However, anxiety can be an unwanted side effect[44] of using cannabis that can result from too high a dose, the wrong cannabis varietal, or simply the placebo effect[45] of hearing marijuana can cause anxiety. Certain molecules in cannabis like CBD definitely decrease anxiety.[46]

Arthritis

The active ingredients in cannabis have been shown in cell and animal[47] studies[48] [49] as well as human clinical trials[50] and in patient self-reports to ease the inflammation[51] of rheumatoid arthritis and the perception of pain in osteoarthritis. Both actions can reduce the patient's sensation of arthritis pain, and arthritis is one of the leading causes of becoming a medical cannabis patient, according to state and country-level data.

Nausea/Appetite/Wasting

Increased appetite is considered by the American Medical Association to be an "adverse effect" of taking cannabis, but for many, that is the chief goal. The active ingredients in cannabis have been shown in cell and animal studies[52] [53] as well as human clinical trials[54] and in patient self-reports[55] to decrease nausea[56], and bring on appetite, which can help stave off the wasting associated with a wide variety of conditions, including cancer, HIV/AIDS, and Alzheimer's disease.

Crohn's Disease

The active ingredients in cannabis have been shown in cell and animal studies[57] as well as human clinical trials[58] and in patient self-reports to dampen a body's overactive immune system. Left unchecked, your immune system can tear apart your body's nerves and other tissues, and lead to death. Crohn's disease is a painful bowel disorder caused by immune system-related inflammation[59] in the gut. Patients use cannabis products to reduce the nausea, pain, and cramping of Crohn's disease.

Cancer[60]

The modern medical cannabis age got underway because a cancer patient reported cannabis provided relief from chemotherapy nausea. Among the 23 medical cannabis states, cancer is a leading qualifying condition. The active ingredients in cannabis have been shown[61] in cell and animal studies as well as a few human trials[62] [63] and in patient self-reports to ease the nausea[64] and wasting[65] [66] associated with cancer and chemotherapy, plus help treat insomnia and depression.

Evidence is also accumulating[67] that cannabis not only offers relief from the symptoms of cancer, but may also encourage the destruction of cancer cells. Cell[68] and animal studies[69] and small experimental human trials[70] [71] have confirmed[72] that the active ingredients in cannabis may stop certain types of cancer from growing[73], cause cancer cells to commit suicide, and block cancer cells' acquisition of new blood supplies.[74]

Hepatitis C

Hepatitis C is a virus that can replicate for decades in patients until it causes liver disease or liver cancer, and ultimately death. Hepatitis C is a common qualifying condition for using cannabis, and some of the active ingredients in cannabis have been shown in cell[75] and animal studies[76] as well as human studies[77] and in patient self-reports to slow and stop the replication of Hepatitis C, dampen Hepatitis C-related liver inflammation[78], discourage liver cancer development, and encourage patient sleep and appetite[79].

Glaucoma

One of the oldest, most credible uses for medical cannabis involves its use to treat dangerous pressure in the eye, which causes glaucoma and blindness. Despite its federal illegality, the United States gives out supplies of medical cannabis to a select group of patients, one of whom has glaucoma so bad she would otherwise go blind[80]. The active ingredients in cannabis have been shown in cell and animal studies and in patient self-reports[81] [82] [83] to reduce blood pressure, and in the right doses, intra-ocular blood pressure.

HIV/AIDS

At the dawn of the modern medical cannabis era, HIV and AIDS patients in California were among the first to report medical cannabis helped them live longer, better lives with the disease. Today, we know the active ingredients in cannabis have been shown in cell and animal studies[84] [85] as well as human clinical trials[86] and in patient self-reports to not only fight the nausea[87], wasting, insomnia and depression[88] of HIV/AIDS infection, but make the body less hospitable to the virus itself[89]. Cannabis' active ingredients dampen immune system and inflammatory responses that the HIV/AIDS virus would otherwise hijack in order to better replicate.

Other common indications for medical cannabis

Insomnia

One of the leading indications for cannabis is sleep improvement.[90] Cell, animal, and human trials have all confirmed one of the effects of cannabis can be drowsiness[91]. Cannabis may work on insomnia a number of ways, by reducing pain, anxiety, and muscle tension that are interfering with sleep.

Depression

Depression is another very prominent reason patients report using medical cannabis.[92] Animal and human trials confirm that the primary active ingredient in cannabis, THC, causes euphoria, or feelings of well-being[93], as well as decreases in attention to negative stimuli. Cannabis may also help ease depression by relieving related symptoms like insomnia, lack of appetite[94], pain and anxiety.

Anger/Agitation

Patients report using medical cannabis use to prevent anger[95], and animal and human trials confirm the plant's active ingredients could help control anger by dampening the nervous system's response to negative stimuli, as well as causing feelings of well-being, or euphoria.

Spinal cord damage

Many states allow people with spinal cord damage to use medical cannabis. Cell animal and human studies[96] show[97] that the active ingredients in cannabis interact with nerves in the spinal cord to protect nerve cells during injury and encourage their regrowth, and reduce pain and inflammation.

PTSD

Controversial for some, the science is sound[98] [99] — the molecular root of PTSD can be altered with the active ingredients in marijuana. The result for some is better sleep, fewer nightmares, less daytime agitation, and over time, promoted healing of the brain.

Tourette's Syndrome

Pre-clinical data supports[100] and select human trials find that the main active ingredient in cannabis, THC, was an effective treatment for the tics of Tourette's syndrome.[101] Taking cannabis might also improve certain speech abilities.[102] The bigger the dose, the bigger the effect.[103]

Amyotrophic Lateral Sclerosis[104]

Cannabis protects nerve cells[105] from the damage of ALS and treats the pain and cramps of the disease.[106] Pre-clinical data[107] shows[108] that cannabis modulates the body's main signaling system for motor function and pain, which probably explains why some ALS patients report it helps.

Alzheimer's Disease[109] [110]

Caregivers are using cannabis to treat the agitation and insomnia from Alzheimer's-related dementia[111]. Long-term cannabidiol treatment may slow or stop the progression[112] [113] of Alzheimer's, animal models suggest.[114] [115]

Asthma

Both THC and CBD[116] play a role in decreasing the inflammation of asthma,[117] which is why cannabis has been used for thousands of years as a folk remedy for asthma.

Other less common indications

Ulcerative Colitis/Inflammatory Bowel Disease

Sufferers from this painful bowel disorder report[118] relief using cannabis, and cell[119] and animal[120] [121] and human trials have found the active ingredients in the plant can decrease sensations of pain, as well as regulate the inflammation and immune response sometimes causing the condition.

Type 1 and Type 2 Diabetes

Cell and animal[122] studies as well as limited human trials show the active ingredients in cannabis can beneficially alter[123] the function[124] of the body's insulin system, which is central to the disease of diabetes. Cannabis users tend to be thinner, with less incidence[125] of diabetes[126], than non-users.[127] Diabetic neuropathy is also an indication for cannabis with a lot of supporting evidence.[128] [129]

Huntington's Disease

Thankfully rare, Huntington's disease involves the progressive breakdown of nerve cells in the brain, resulting in movement and thinking deficits. It's incurable. Researchers[130] are looking at the active ingredients in marijuana for Huntington's disease[131] because they protect nerve cells[132] [133]. Cannabis can also provide related symptom relief for sleep disturbance, depression, anxiety and the side effects of other drugs.

Parkinson's Disease[132]

The second most common active ingredient in cannabis, CBD, significantly reduced the agitation of psycho-sis from Parkinson's disease[135] and improved Parkinson's-related sleep disorders in small trials.[136] [137]

Sickle Cell Disease

Cell, animal models[138] and patient reports[139] support the use of cannabis's active ingredients to not only treat the pain and inflammation of sickle cell disease, but to help slow its progression. A limited human trial of inhaled whole-plant cannabis for sickle cell disease is underway in California.

Severe Fibromyaglia

Researchers think this mysterious chronic pain syndrome could be related to dysfunction in the body's nerve signaling system[140] that cannabis can help clear up. Fibromyalgia patients report using it, and limited trials[141] support[142] its use for pain and muscle stiffness.

Traumatic Brain Injury & Post-Concussive Syndrome

The active ingredients in cannabis protect brain cells and help them heal when damaged.[143 144 145] Cannabis is being investigated by researchers and used by patients as an alternative therapy for traumatic brain injuries and post-concussion syndrome. The U.S. government also holds a patent[146] on cannabis' ingredient for use in treating brain damage.

Muscular Dystrophy

The hereditary disease of weakening and wasting muscle, or its symptoms[147], may be treated by cannabis, researchers think.[148] Animal studies[149] support the belief that cannabis helps with muscle spasticity.

ADD/ADHD

Almost as controversial as the diagnosis of attention deficit disorder and the widespread rise in medication for the new disorder is the use of medical cannabis to treat it. Medical cannabis for attention and hyperactivity disorder is supported by a large volume of patient self-reports[150] as well as pre-clinical studies[151] that show the drug affects the same nerve signaling system involved in ADD and ADHD.

Autism/Asperger's

Patients are reporting the use of cannabis to manage symptoms[152] related to autism and Asperger's syndrome, including agitation, and tics. Cell and animal studies[153] indicate the diseases are tied to the functioning of a cell signaling system[154] that cannabis interacts with.

Eczema/Psoriasis

Patients report using cannabis and its extracts — especially topical ointments — as an alternative treatment for chronic incurable eczema and psoriasis — conditions that are often related to immune system function. Cannabis can suppress an overactive immune system. Cell and animal studies also support the use of cannabinoids for such conditions.[155 156 157 158 159]

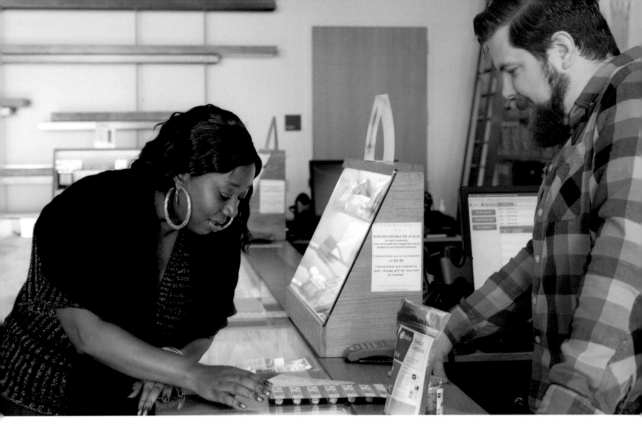

Pre-Menstrual Syndrome

Cannabis is known to treat many of the symptoms associated with pre-menstrual syndrome, especially pain, cramping, and anxiety, but not fatigue. Cannabis' active ingredients interact with a major cell signaling system throughout the human reproductive system. [160]

Senile Dementia/Agitation

At the right doses, cannabis can sedate and calm patients with senile dementia and agitation[161]. The active ingredients in the plant also appear to protect against the progression of degenerative brain disease.[162]

Doctor's "Recommendation" NOT "Prescription"

In the United States, doctors do not write a "prescription" for cannabis, they write a "recommendation." The difference is a very important legal distinction that protects doctors from prosecution for violating federal drug control laws.

Under federal law, cannabis is classified as among the most dangerous, medically useless drugs on the planet, alongside heroin, LSD, mescaline (peyote), and ecstasy.

Doctors are not allowed to "prescribe" such drugs. However, under the First Amendment of the Constitution of the United States, doctors have the right to free speech, and that speech can include "recommending" cannabis to a patient. This distinction is federal law under the case Conant v. Walters.[163]

The difference may seem like semantics, but these semantics are what allows medical cannabis to be widely available by "recommendation" in California and other states, yet still be banned in places like the South where there are laws mandating a "prescription" for cannabis.

Obtaining a doctor's recommendation can be a quick or lengthy process depending on state law and doctor.

In places like California with simple rules, a doctor can qualify a patient via a teleconference interview.

By contrast, some CBD-only programs in the Midwest, East and South require finding a specialist at a specific hospital, developing a year-long doctor-patient relationship, and providing reams of medical records — all to enter a very limited clinical trial.

Generally, most recommendation visits will occur at a cannabis clinic by appointment or walk-in, and involve some standard medical history forms to fill out, an in-person interview and exam.

Bringing in past medical records confirming qualifying conditions (like cancer) is always useful, no matter which state.

At the end, the doctor gives you a signed, dated recommendation that qualifies you as a patient, or goes into your application packet for a state's program.

For more on finding a cannabis-specialized clinician, see Resources.

State ID Card

Patients often use the word "card," "medical card" or "marijuana card" to refer to their basic doctor's recommendation for medical cannabis. These recommendations often come in written form, with an ID-card-sized recommendation for carrying around in your wallet.

A wallet-signed recommendation from a doctor is different than an official state medical marijuana identification card, which usually requires more paperwork, and usually comes with more rights.

The stricter a state's medical marijuana system, the more lengthy and expensive is the process to obtain an ID card. However, states with these strict systems also often provide card-

holders with immunity from arrest for certain marijuana crimes like possession or use. Without a card, a qualified patient can often still be arrested, transported to jail, held, released, and arraigned. Only then does a patient get what's called an "affirmative defense" for legal use of medical marijuana. An affirmative defense is merely a shield in court. A registration card is a shield on the street.

Check with the State-By-State Guide to see if you need or want a registration card, and expect to fill out some forms akin to a driver's license or concealed handgun permit.

You will almost always have to include your doctor's recommendation, and some states make doctors do the applying for you.

You're going to need to prove residency, have valid contact information like a home and email address, and a Social Security Number.

Many programs will check your background and disqualify you or a caregiver for certain convictions. Some programs will require you submit a full set of fingerprints for an FBI background check.

Most of these registration card programs come with substantial fees ($75-$200), have waivers for the poor, and require annual renewal. When you get the card, you keep it on your person, use it to get access to dispensaries, and to avoid arrest for certain marijuana crimes.

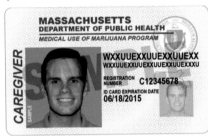

Sources of Legal Medical Cannabis

> "Cannabis therapeutics is personalized medicine. One size doesn't fit all with respect to cannabis therapeutics, and neither does one compound or one product or one strain."
>
> — Martin A. Lee, director of Project CBD, author of *Smoke Signals: A Social History of Marijuana — Medical, Recreational and Scientific*

With a doctor's recommendation and registry ID card (if mandatory), you are ready to legally acquire cannabis. Many states have limits on how much you can possess or grow, usually a few ounces of dried flowers, or a few mature plants, and you'll want to stay under those limits.

Public Dispensary

By far the easiest and most practical way to obtain medical cannabis is to go into a store and buy it, if such places are legal in your state and are nearby.

Places like California have several thousand dispensaries that are not yet licensed by the state, but are licensed at the city and county level. By contrast, in tightly controlled medical cannabis regimes found on the East Coast, there might be just one state-licensed dispensary available for the entire state. CBD-only states generally lack any such dispensaries.

Private Collective

Some less restrictive medical cannabis states allow for private collectives or cooperatives of patients and their caregivers to grow and share medical cannabis. Private collectives are more difficult to locate than publicly listed dispensaries, with a smaller selection and unique hours or modes of operation.

In an easy-access states like California, Colorado, Washington and Oregon, private collectives are very popular — especially ones that deliver.

Caregiver

Most medical marijuana states make an allowance for a "caregiver" to either obtain and transport, or grow cannabis for a patient or patients. Caregivers often have to be at least 18 or 21 years of age. Some states allow one caregiver to have multiple patients. Other states mandate one patient per caregiver. If the patient is a minor, their parent or guardian is often a required caregiver.

Designating someone as a caregiver can be as easy as an oral agreement (California) or as hard as turning in a separate caregiver application to the state, with copy of passport-style photo, full fingerprints, background check and $100 fee.

Self-Grow

Depending on your state law, you may be able to legally grow cannabis for yourself, or have a caregiver do it.

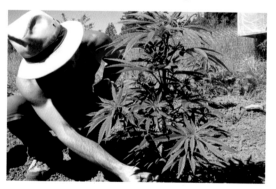

Growing is often limited to a few plants and subject to rules for security and access. Medical growing can also be legal at the state level, and still subject to local bans, as in California and elsewhere. It's not easy to grow medical-grade cannabis. It requires seeds or clones, security, appropriate temperature, humidity, light, water, nutrients and sanitation, and several months of regular gardening.

Illegal Market

The United States extremely underserves its medical cannabis patients, while at the same time maintains a failed prohibition on marijuana for recreational use. The result is that the people who objectively need cannabis the most (say, elderly hospice patients) have the least access to it, compared to the average American teenager.

This book is about ways to legally obtain medical cannabis, so we don't go into how to illegally obtain marijuana, but we will say that doing so is probably more popular than all the legal ways, combined.

Just a tiny fraction of the nation are qualified patients — with access to dispensaries, collectives, home-growing, or a caregiver. By contrast, about half the nation is estimated to have tried marijuana, and about 6 percent of the U.S. population uses it daily or near-daily.[164]

Marijuana use by age generally peaks in the early 20s. Most 10th grade high school students have consistently reported for decades in national drug surveys that marijuana is either "easy" or "very easy" to obtain in their communities.[165]

When it's a matter of life and death, breaking the law to score some pot is far less of a risk than going without.

A person is statistically likely to be arrested for marijuana about once per 10 years of daily use.[166]

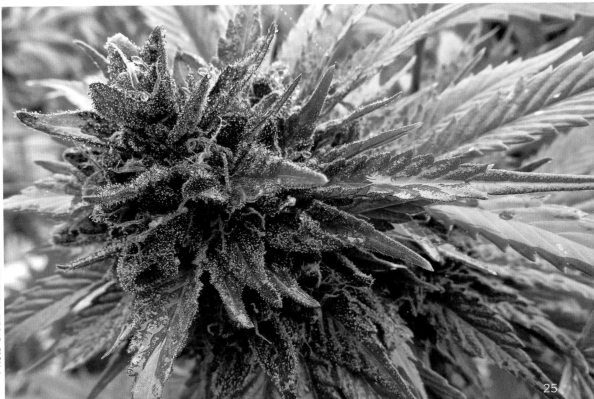

Photo Credit: David Downs

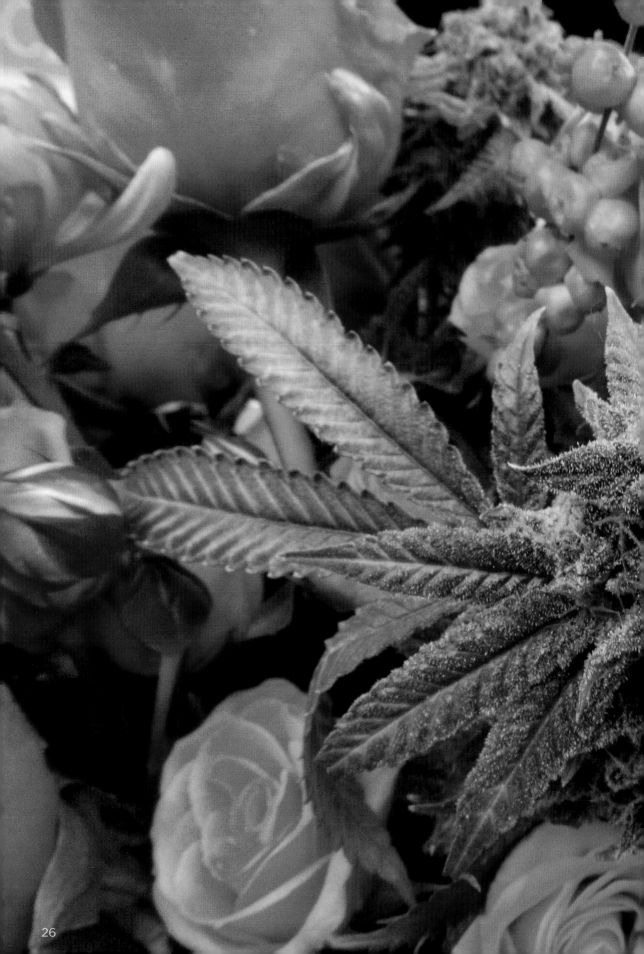

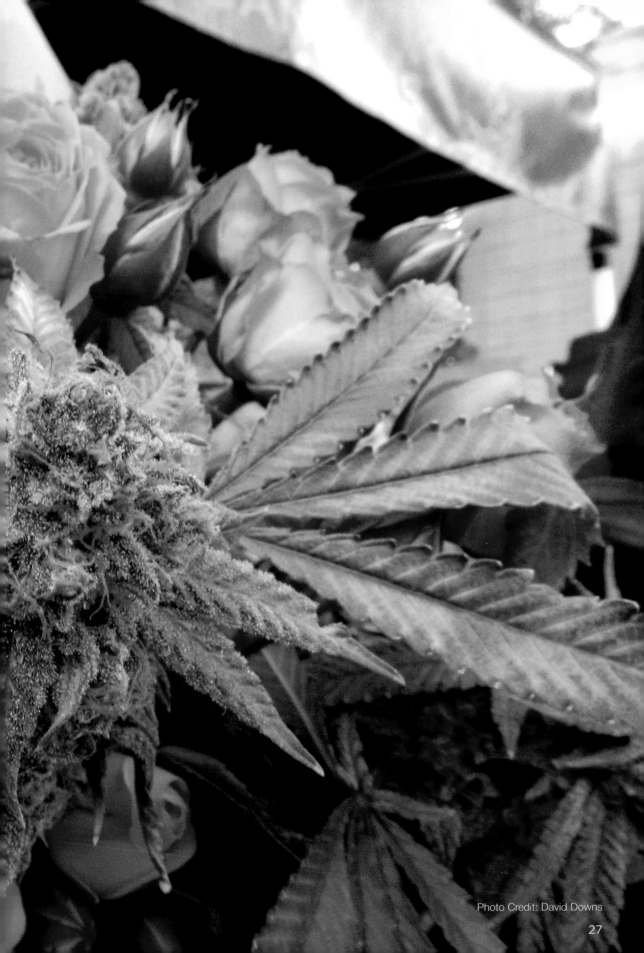

Photo Credit: David Downs

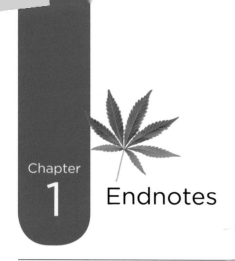

Chapter 1 Endnotes

1 Abrams, Dr. Donald, 2014, interview.

2 Reiman, Amanda, Cannabis as a substitute for alcohol and other drugs. Harm Reduction Journal. 2009, 6:35. doi:10.1186/1477-7517-6-35.

3 Nunberg H, Kilmer B, Pacula RL, Burgdorf J. An Analysis of Applicants Presenting to a Medical Marijuana Specialty Practice in California. Journal of drug policy analysis. 2011;4(1):1. doi:10.2202/1941-2851.1017.

4 Arizona Dept of Health Services report, 2014: AZDHS.gov, http://azdhs.gov/documents/preparedness/medical-marijuana/reports/2014/arizona-medical-marijuana-end-of-year-report-2014.pdf.

5 Thompson AE. Medical Marijuana. JAMA 2015;313(24):2508. doi:10.1001/jama.2015.6676.

6 Russo, EB. 2001. Handbook of psychotropic herbs: A scientific analysis of herbal remedies for psychiatric conditions. Binghamton, NY: Haworth Press. Hemp for headache: An in-depth historical and scientific review of cannabis in migraine treatment. J Cannabis Therapeutics 1 (2):21-92.

7 Zaller N, Topletz A, Frater S, Yates G, Lally M. Profiles of medicinal cannabis patients attending compassion centers in rhode island. J Psychoactive Drugs. 2015 Jan-Mar;47(1):18-23. doi: 10.1080/02791072.2014.999901.

8 Wilsey B, Marcotte T, Tsodikov A, et al. A randomized, placebo-controlled, crossover trial of cannabis cigarettes in neuropathic pain. Journal of Pain 2008;9:506-521.

9 Wilsey B, Marcotte T, Deutsch R, et al. Low-dose vaporized cannabis significantly improves neuropathic pain. Journal of Pain 2012;14:136-148.

10 Hill KP. Medical Marijuana for Treatment of Chronic Pain and Other Medical and Psychiatric Problems: A Clinical Review. JAMA. 2015;313(24):2474-2483. doi:10.1001/jama.2015.6199.

11 Lynch ME, Campbell F. Cannabinoids for treatment of chronic non-cancer pain; a systematic

review of randomized trials. Br J Clin Pharmacol. 2011;72:735-744.

12 Abrams DI, Vizoso HP, Shade SB, et al. Vaporization as a smokeless cannabis delivery system: A pilot study. Clin Pharmacol Ther. 2007;82:572-578.

13 Wallace M, Schulteis G, Atkinson JH, et al. Dose-dependent effects of smoked cannabis on capsaicin-induced pain and hyperalgesia in healthy volunteers. Anesthesiology 2007;107:785-796.

14 Martin-Sanchez E, Furukawa TA, Taylor J, Martin JLR. Systematic review and metaanalysis of cannabis treatment for chronic pain. Pain Medicine 2009;10;1353-1368.

15 Whiting PF, Wolff RF, Deshpande S, et al. Cannabinoids for Medical Use: A Systematic Review and Meta-analysis. JAMA. 2015;313(24):2456-2473. doi:10.1001/jama.2015.6358.

16 Abrams DI, Couey P, Shade SB, et al. Cannabinoid-opioid interaction in chronic pain. Clin Pharmacol Ther. 2011:90;844-851.

17 Rog DJ, Nurmikko TJ, Friede T, Young CA. Randomized, controlled trial of cannabis-based medicine in central pain in multiple sclerosis. Neurology 2005;65:812-819.

18 Abrams DI, Jay CA, Shade SB, et al. Cannabis in painful HIV-associated sensory neuropathy: A randomized placebo-controlled trial. Neurology 2007;68:515-521.

19 Lynch, M.E., Ware, Mark A. Cannabinoids for the Treatment of Chronic Non-Cancer Pain: An Updated Systematic Review of Randomized Controlled Trials . J Neuroimmune Pharmacol (2015) 10:293–301 DOI 10.1007/s11481-015-9600-6

20 Bachhuber MA, Saloner B, Cunningham CO, Barry CL. Medical Cannabis Laws and Opioid Analgesic Overdose Mortality in the United States, 1999-2010. JAMA Intern Med. 2014;174(10):1668-1673. doi:10.1001/jamainternmed.2014.4005.

21 Tongtong Wang, MSc, Jean-Paul Collet, PhD MD, Stan Shapiro, PhD, and Mark A. Ware, MBBS MSc Adverse effects of medical cannabinoids: a systematic review CMAJ June 17, 2008; 178:1669-1678; doi:10.1503/cmaj.071178.

22 Zajicek JP, Fox P, Sanders H, et al; UK MS Research Group. Cannabinoids for treatment of spasticity and other symptoms related to multiple sclerosis (CAMS study): multicentre randomised placebo-controlled trial. Lancet 2003;362:1517-1526.

23 Vaney C, Heinzel-Gutenbrunner M, Jobin P, et al. Efficacy, safety and tolerability of an orally administered cannabis extract in the treatment of spasticity in patients with multiple sclerosis: a randomized, double-blind, placebo-controlled, crossover study. Mult Scler 2004;10:417-424.

24 Wade DT, Makela P, Robson P, et al. Do cannabis-based medicinal extracts have general or specific effects on symptoms in multiple sclerosis? A double-blind, randomized, placebo-controlled study on 160 patients. Mult Scler 2004;10:434-441.

25 Hill KP. Medical Marijuana for Treatment of Chronic Pain and Other Medical and Psychiatric Problems: A Clinical Review. JAMA. 2015;313(24):2474-2483. doi:10.1001/jama.2015.6199.

26 Whiting PF, Wolff RF, Deshpande S, et al. Cannabinoids for Medical Use: A Systematic Review and Meta-analysis. JAMA. 2015;313(24):2456-2473. doi:10.1001/jama.2015.6358.

27 Nagarkatti P, Pandey R, Rieder SA, Hegde VL, Nagarkatti M. Cannabinoids as novel anti-inflammatory drugs. Future medicinal chemistry. 2009;1(7):1333-1349. doi:10.4155/fmc.09.93.

28 Gloss D, Vickrey B. Cannabinoids for epilepsy. Cochrane Database of Systematic Reviews 2014, Issue 3. Art. No.:CD009270.

29 Gloss D, Vickrey B. Cannabinoids for epilepsy. Cochrane Database of Systematic Reviews 2014, Issue 3. Art. No.:CD009270.

30 Wallace, MJ, et al. 2003. The endogenous cannabinoid system regulates seizure frequency and duration in a model of temporal lobe epilepsy. J Pharmacol Exp Ther 307 (1):129-37.

31 RG dos Santos PhD, JEC Hallak MD PhD, JP Leite MD PhD, AW Zuardi MD PhD, JAS Crippa MD PhD. Phytocannabinoids and epilepsy, Journal of Clinical Pharmacy and Therapeutics, 2015, 40, 135–143. doi: 10.1111/jcpt.12235.

32 Porter, BE, Jacobson, C. Report of a parent survey of cannabidiol-enriched cannabis use in pediatric treatment-resistant epilepsy. Epilepsy & Behavior 2013;29:574-577.

33 Lorenz, R. 2004. On the application of cannabis in paediatrics and epileptology. Neuroendocrinol Lett 25 (1-2):40-44.

34 Porter, BE & Jacobson, C. (2013). Report of a parent survey of cannabidiol-enriched cannabis use in

pediatric treatment-resistant epilepsy. Epilepsy Behav, 29, 574-7.

35 Hussain SA, Zhou R, Jacobson C, Weng J, Cheng E, Lay J, Hung P, Lerner JT, Sankar R. Perceived efficacy of cannabidiol-enriched cannabis extracts for treatment of pediatric epilepsy: A potential role for infantile spasms and Lennox-Gastaut syndrome. Epilepsy Behav. 2015 Jun;47:138-41. doi: 10.1016/j.yebeh.2015.04.009.

36 Press CA, Knupp KG, Chapman KE. Parental reporting of response to oral cannabis extracts for treatment of refractory epilepsy. Epilepsy Behav. 2015 Apr;45:49-52. doi: 10.1016/j.yebeh.2015.02.043.

37 Bradstreet, James Jeffrey. Understanding Cannabinoids and Epilepsy, Brain Treatment Center of Atlanta, Western University of Health Sciences.

38 Cunha JM, Carlini EA, Pereira AE, Ramos OL, Pimentel C, Gagliardi R, Sanvito WL, Lander N, Mechoulam R. Chronic administration of cannabidiol to healthy volunteers and epileptic patients. Pharmacology. 1980;21(3):175-85. PubMed PMID: 7413719.

39 RG dos Santos PhD, JEC Hallak MD PhD, JP Leite MD PhD, AW Zuardi MD PhD, JAS Crippa MD PhD. Phytocannabinoids and epilepsy, Journal of Clinical Pharmacy and Therapeutics, 2015; 40, 135–143. doi: 10.1111/jcpt.12235.

40 Moreira FA, Wotjak CT. Cannabinoids and anxiety. Curr Top Behav Neurosci. 2010;2:429-50. Review. PubMed PMID: 21309120.

41 Crippa JA, Derenusson GN, Ferrari TB, Wichert-Ana L, Duran FL, Martin-Santos R, Simões MV, Bhattacharyya S, Fusar-Poli P, Atakan Z, Santos Filho A, Freitas-Ferrari MC, McGuire PK, Zuardi AW, Busatto GF, Hallak JE. Neural basis of anxiolytic effects of cannabidiol (CBD) in generalized social anxiety disorder: a preliminary report. J Psychopharmacol. 2011 Jan;25(1):121-30. doi:10.1177/0269881110379283.

42 Nunberg H, Kilmer B, Pacula RL, Burgdorf J. An Analysis of Applicants Presenting to a Medical Marijuana Specialty Practice in California. Journal of drug policy analysis. 2011;4(1):1. doi:10.2202/1941-2851.1017.

43 Whiting PF, Wolff RF, Deshpande S, et al. Cannabinoids for Medical Use: A Systematic Review and Meta-analysis. JAMA. 2015;313(24):2456-2473. doi:10.1001/jama.2015.6358.

44 Metrik J, Aston ER, Kahler CW, Rohsenow DJ, Knopik VS. Marijuana's Acute Effects on Cognitive Bias for Affective and Marijuana Cues. Exp Clin Psychopharmacol. 2015 Jul 13. [Epub ahead of print] PubMed PMID: 26167716.

45 Backes, Michael. Cannabis Pharmacy. 2014. Black Dog & Leventhal, New York. Pg. 36.

46 Bergamaschi MM, Queiroz RH, Chagas MH, et al. Cannabidiol reduces the anxiety induced by simulated public speaking in treatment-naïve social phobia patients. Neuropsychopharmacology 2011; 36(6): 1219-26.

47 Schuelert N, McDougall JJ. Cannabinoid-mediated antinociception is enhanced in rat osteoarthritic knees. Arthritis Rheum 2008;58:145–53.

48 Fukuda S, Kohsaka H, Takayasu A, Yokoyama W, Miyabe C, Miyabe Y, Harigai M, Miyasaka N, Nanki T. Cannabinoid receptor 2 as a potential therapeutic target in rheumatoid arthritis. BMC Musculoskelet Disord. 2014 Aug 12;15:275. doi:10.1186/1471-2474-15-275. PubMed PMID: 25115332; PubMed Central PMCID:PMC4243420.

49 La Porta C, Bura SA, Negrete R, Maldonado R. Involvement of the endocannabinoid system in osteoarthritis pain. Eur J Neurosci. 2014 Feb;39(3):485-500. doi:10.1111/ejn.12468.

50 Blake DR, Robson P, Ho M, Jubb RW, McCabe CS. Preliminary assessment of the efficacy, tolerability and safety of a cannabis-based medicine (Sativex) in the treatment of pain caused by rheumatoid arthritis. Rheumatology. January 2006 45 (1): 50-52 first published online Nov. 9, 2005; doi:10.1093/rheumatology/kei183.

51 Nagarkatti P, Pandey R, Rieder SA, Hegde VL, Nagarkatti M. Cannabinoids as novel anti-inflammatory drugs. Future medicinal chemistry. 2009;1(7):1333-1349. doi:10.4155/fmc.09.93.

52 Mechoulam R, Berry EM, Avraham Y, et al.: Endocannabinoids, feeding and suckling--from our perspective. Int J Obes (Lond) 30 (Suppl 1): S24-8, 2006.

53 Koch JE. Delta(9)-THC stimulates food intake in Lewis rats: effects on chow, high-fat and sweet high-fat diets. Pharmacol Biochem Behav 2001; 68: 539–43.

54 Whiting PF, Wolff RF, Deshpande S, et al. Cannabinoids for Medical

Use: A Systematic Review and Meta-analysis. JAMA. 2015;313(24):2456-2473. doi:10.1001/jama.2015.6358.

55 Nunberg H, Kilmer B, Pacula RL, Burgdorf J. An Analysis of Applicants Presenting to a Medical Marijuana Specialty Practice in California. Journal of drug policy analysis. 2011;4(1):1. doi:10.2202/1941-2851.1017.

56 Thompson AE. Medical Marijuana. JAMA. 2015;313(24):2508. doi:10.1001/jama.2015.6676.

57 Massa F, Monory K. Endocannabinoids and the gastrointestinal tract. J Endocrinol Invest. 2006;29(3 Suppl):47-57. Review. PubMed PMID: 16751708.

58 Naftali T, Bar-Lev Schleider L, Dotan I, Lansky EP, Sklerovsky Benjaminov F, Konikoff FM. Cannabis induces a clinical response in patients with Crohn's disease: a prospective placebo-controlled study. Clin Gastroenterol Hepatol. 2013 Oct;11(10):1276-1280.e1. doi: 10.1016/j.cgh.2013.04.034 Epub 2013 May 4. PubMed PMID: 23648372.

59 Nagarkatti P, Pandey R, Rieder SA, Hegde VL, Nagarkatti M. Cannabinoids as novel anti-inflammatory drugs. Future medicinal chemistry. 2009;1(7):1333-1349. doi:10.4155/fmc.09.93.

60 Minnesota Health Dept., A Review of Medical Cannabis Studies relating to Chemical Compositions and Dosages for Qualifying Medical Conditions, Dec. 2014, http://www.health.state.mn.us/topics/cannabis/practitioners/dosage.pdf.

61 Tramer MR, Carroll D, Campbell FA, et al. Cannabinoids for control of chemotherapy-induced nausea and vomiting: quantitative systematic review. BMJ 2001;323:16-21.

62 Musty R, Rossi R. Effects of smoked cannabis and oral delta-9-tetrahydrocannabinol on nausea and emesis after cancer chemotherapy: A review of state clinical trials. Journal of Cannabis Therapeutics 2001;1:29-42.

63 Machado Rocha FC, Stefano SC, De Cassia Haiek R, et al. Therapeutic use of Cannabis sativa on chemotherapy-induced nausea and vomiting among cancer patients: systematic review and meta-analysis. Eur J Cancer Care 2008;17:431-443.

64 Chang AE, Shiling DJ, Stillman RC, et al.: Delta-9-tetrahydrocannabinol as an antiemetic in cancer patients receiving high-dose metho-

trexate. A prospective, randomized evaluation. Ann Intern Med 91 (6): 819-24, 1979.

65 Nelson K, Walsh D, Deeter P, Sheehan F. A phase II study of delta-9-tetrahydrocannabinol for appetite stimulation in cancer-associated anorexia. J Palliat Care 1994;10:14-18.

66 Mantovani G, Maccio A, Madeddu C, et al. Randomized phase III clinical trial of five different arms of treatment in 332 patients with cancer cachexia. Oncologist 2010;15:200-211.

67 Sarafaraz et al. 2008. Cannabinoids for cancer treatment: progress and promise. Cancer Research 68: 339-342.

68 Vaccani A, Massi P, Parolaro D. 2003. Inhibition of human glioma cell growth by the nonpsychoactive cannabidiol. Paper read at First European Workshop on Cannabinoid Research, April 4-5, at Madrid.

69 cancer.gov, 2015. NCIPDQCAM, Cannabis and Cannabinoids-for health professionals (PDQ), http://www.cancer.gov/about-cancer/treatment/cam/hp/cannabis-pdq#link/_26_toc.

70 Velasco G, Sánchez C, Guzmán M: Toward the use of cannabinoids as anti-tumour agents. Nat Rev Cancer 12 (6): 436-44, 2012.

71 Guzmán M, Duarte MJ, Blázquez C, et al.: A pilot clinical study of Delta9-tetrahydrocannabinol in patients with recurrent glioblastoma multiforme. Br J Cancer 95 (2): 197-203, 2006.

72 Werner, Clint. Marijuana - Gateway to Health, 2011, Dachstar Press.

73 Nagarkatti P, Pandey R, Rieder SA, Hegde VL, Nagarkatti M. Cannabinoids as novel anti-inflammatory drugs. Future medicinal chemistry. 2009;1(7):1333-1349. doi:10.4155/fmc.09.93.

74 Werner, Clint. Marijuana - Gateway to Health, 2011, Dachstar Press.

75 Teixeira-Clerc F, Julien B, Grenard P, Tran Van Nhieu J, Deveaux V, Hezode C, Mallat A, Lotersztajn S. [The endocannabinoid system as a novel target for the treatment of liver fibrosis]. Pathol Biol (Paris). 2008 Feb;56(1):36-8. Epub 2007 Apr 6. Review. French. PubMed PMID: 17412522.

76 Baldassarre M, Giannone FA, Napoli L, Tovoli A, Ricci CS, Tufoni M, Caraceni P. The endocannabinoid system in advanced liver cirrhosis: pathophysiological implication and future perspectives. Liver Int. 2013 Oct;33(9):1298-308. doi: 10.1111/liv.12263. Epub 2013 Jul 25. Review. PubMed PMID: 23890208.

77 Caraceni P, Domenicali M, Giannone F, Bernardi M. The role of the endocannabinoid system in liver diseases. Best Pract Res Clin Endocrinol Metab. 2009 Feb;23(1):65-77. doi: 10.1016/j.beem.2008.10.009. Review. PubMed PMID: 19285261.

78 Nagarkatti P, Pandey R, Rieder SA, Hegde VL, Nagarkatti M. Cannabinoids as novel anti-inflammatory drugs. Future medicinal chemistry. 2009;1(7):1333-1349. doi:10.4155/fmc.09.93.

79 Backes. Cannabis Pharmacy, 2014. pg. 207.

80 Federal Compassionate Investigational New Drug program.

81 Jarvinen T, Pate D, Laine K. 2002. Cannabinoids in the treatment of glaucoma. Pharmacol Ther 95 (2):203.

82 Tomida I, Pertwee RG, zuara-Blanco A. Cannabinoids and glaucoma. Br J Ophthalmol. 2004;88:708-713.

83 Wan MJ, Daniel S, Kassam F, et al. Survey of complementary and alternative medicine use in glaucoma patients. J Glaucoma 2012;21:79-82.

84 Chandra LC, Kumar V, Torben W, Vande Stouwe C, Winsauer P, Amedee A, Molina PE, Mohan M. Chronic administration of 9-tetrahydrocannabinol induces intestinal anti-inflammatory microRNA expression during acute simian immunodeficiency virus infection of rhesus macaques. J Virol. 2015 Jan 15;89(2):1168-81. doi: 10.1128/JVI.01754-14. Epub 2014 Nov 5. PubMed PMID: 25378491; PubMed Central PMCID: PMC4300675.

85 Molina et al. 2011. Cannabinoid administration attenuates the progression of simian immunodeficiency virus. AIDS Research and Human Retroviruses 27: 585-592.

86 Abrams DI, Hilton JF, Leiser RJ, et al. Short-term effects of cannabinoids in patients with HIV-1 infection; a randomized, placebo-controlled clinical trial. Ann Intern Med 2003;139:258-266.

87 Haney M, Gunderson EW, Rabkin J, et al. Dronabinol and marijuana in HIV-positive marijuana smokers: Caloric intake, mood, and sleep. J Acquir Immune Defic Syndr. 2007;45:545-554.

88 Haney M, Rabkin J, Gunderson E, Foltin RW. Dronabinol and marijuana in HIV(+) marijuana smokers: acute effects on caloric intake and mood. Psychopharmacology 2005;181:170-178.

89 Milloy MJ, Marshall B, Kerr T, Richardson L, Hogg R, Guillemi S, Montaner JS, Wood E. High-intensity cannabis use associated with lower plasma human immunodeficiency virus-1 RNA viral load among recently infected people who use injection drugs. Drug Alcohol Rev. 2015 Mar;34(2):135-40. doi: 10.1111/dar.12223.

90 Nunberg H, Kilmer B, Pacula RL, Burgdorf J. An Analysis of Applicants Presenting to a Medical Marijuana Specialty Practice in California. Journal of drug policy analysis. 2011;4(1):1. doi:10.2202/1941-2851.1017.

91 AMA, ibid.

92 Nunberg H, Kilmer B, Pacula RL, Burgdorf J. An Analysis of Applicants Presenting to a Medical Marijuana Specialty Practice in California. Journal of drug policy analysis. 2011;4(1):1. doi:10.2202/1941-2851.1017.

93 AMA, ibid.

94 Koch, et al. Hypothalamic POMC neurons promote cannabinoid-induced feeding. Nature 519, 45–50 (05 March 2015) doi:10.1038/nature14260.

95 Werner, Clint. Marijuana - Gateway to Health, 2011, Dachstar Press.

96 Wade DT, Robson P, House H, Makela P, Aram J. A preliminary controlled study to determine whether whole-plant cannabis extracts can improve intractable neurogenic symptoms. Clin Rehabil. 2003 Feb;17(1):21-9. PubMed PMID: 12617376.

97 Arevalo-Martin A, Molina-Holgado E, Garcia-Ovejero D. Cannabinoids to treat spinal cord injury. Prog Neuropsychopharmacol Biol Psychiatry. 2015 Mar 21. pii: S0278-5846(15)00057-3. doi: 10.1016/j.pnpbp.2015.03.008. [Epub ahead of print] PubMed PMID: 25805333.

98 Jarvinen, T, Pate D, Laine K. 2002. Cannabinoids in the treatment of glaucoma. Pharmacol Ther 95 (2):203.

99 Stern CA, Gazarini L, Vanvossen AC, Zuardi AW, Galve-Roperh I, Guimaraes FS, Takahashi RN, Bertoglio LJ. (9)-Tetrahydrocannabinol alone and combined with cannabidiol mitigate fear memory through reconsolidation disruption. Eur Neuropsychopharmacol. 2015 Jun;25(6):958-65. doi: 10.1016/j.euroneuro.2015.02.001. Epub 2015 Feb 16. PubMed PMID: 25799920.

100 Müller-Vahl KR, Kolbe H, Schneider U, Emrich HM. Cannabis in movement disorders. Forsch Komplementarmed. 1999 Oct;6 Suppl 3:23-7. Review. PubMed PMID: 10627163.

101 Müller-Vahl KR, Schneider U, Prevedel H, Theloe K, Kolbe H, Daldrup T, Emrich HM. Delta 9-tetrahydrocannabinol (THC) is effective in the treatment of tics in Tourette syndrome: a 6-week randomized trial. J Clin Psychiatry. 2003 Apr;64(4):459-65. PubMed PMID: 12716250.

102 Müller-Vahl KR, Prevedel H, Theloe K, Kolbe H, Emrich HM, Schneider U. Treatment of Tourette syndrome with delta-9-tetrahydrocannabinol (delta 9-THC): no influence on neuropsychological performance. Neuropsychopharmacology. 2003 Feb;28(2):384-8. PubMed PMID: 12589392.

103 Müller-Vahl KR, Schneider U, Koblenz A, Jöbges M, Kolbe H, Daldrup T, Emrich HM. Treatment of Tourette's syndrome with Delta 9-tetrahydrocannabinol (THC): a randomized crossover trial. Pharmacopsychiatry. 2002 Mar;35(2):57-61. PubMed PMID: 11951146.

104 Russo, Ethan. Future of Cannabis and Cannabinoids in Therapeutics, Journal of Cannabis Therapeutics, The Haworth Integrative Healing Press. Vol. 3, No. 4, 2003, pp. 163-174.

105 Raman C, McAllister SD, Rizvi G, Patel SG, Moore DH, Abood ME. Amyotrophic lateral sclerosis: delayed disease progression in mice by treatment with a cannabinoid. Amyotroph Lateral Scler Other Motor Neuron Disord. 2004 Mar;5(1):33-9.

106 Joerger M, Wilkins J, Fagagnini S, Baldinger R, Brenneisen R, Schneider U, Goldman B, Weber M. Single-dose pharmacokinetics and tolerability of oral delta-9-tetrahydrocannabinol in patients with amyotrophic lateral sclerosis. Drug Metab Lett. 2012 Jun 1;6(2):102-8. PubMed PMID: 22594565.

107 Carter, et al. 2010. Cannabis and amyotrophic lateral sclerosis: hypothetical and practical applications, and a call for clinical trials. American Journal of Hospice & Palliative Medicine 27: 347-356.

108 Pertwee RG. Targeting the endocannabinoid system with cannabinoid receptor agonists: pharmacological strategies and therapeutic possibilities. Philos Trans R Soc Lond B Biol Sci. 2012 Dec 5;367(1607):3353-63. doi: 10.1098/rstb.2011.0381. Review. PubMed PMID: 23108552; PubMed Central PMCID: PMC3481523.

109 Russo, 2003.

110 Volicer, L, Stelly M, Morris J, McLaughlin J, Volicer BJ. 1997. Effects of dronabinol on anorexia and disturbed behavior in patients with Alzheimer's disease. Int J Geriatr Psychiatry 12 (9):913-9.

111 Walther, et al. 2006. Delta-9-tetrahydrocannabinol for nighttime agitation in severe dementia. Physcopharmacology 185: 524-528.

112 Eubanks, et al. 2006. A molecular link between the active component of marijuana and Alzheimer's disease pathology. Molecular Pharmaceutics 3: 773-777.

113 Ramirez BG, et al. Prevention of Alzheimer's disease pathology by cannabinoids: neuroprotection mediated by blockade of microglial activation. J Neurosci 2005;25(8):1904-13;

114 Cheng D, Spiro AS, Jenner AM, Garner B, Karl T. Long-term cannabidiol treatment prevents the development of social recognition memory deficits in Alzheimer's disease transgenic mice. J Alzheimers Dis. 2014;42(4):1383-96. doi: 10.3233/JAD-140921. PubMed PMID: 25024347.

115 Werner, Clint. Marijuana - Gateway to Health, 2011, Dachstar Press.

116 Koppel BS, Brust JCM, Fife T, et al. Systematic review: Efficacy and safety of medical marijuana in selected neurologic disorders. Neurology 2014;82:1556-1563.

117 Nagarkatti P, Pandey R, Rieder SA, Hegde VL, Nagarkatti M. Cannabinoids as novel anti-inflammatory drugs. Future medicinal chemistry. 2009;1(7):1333-1349. doi:10.4155/fmc.09.93.

118 Jamontt JM, Molleman A, Pertwee RG, Parsons ME. The effects of Delta-tetrahydrocannabinol and cannabidiol alone and in combination on damage, inflammation and

in vitro motility disturbances in rat colitis. Br J Pharmacol. 2010 Jun;160(3):712-23. doi: 10.1111/j.1476-5381.2010.00791.x.

119 Massa F, Marsicano G, Hermann H, Cannich A, Monory K, Cravatt BF, Ferri GL, Sibaev A, Storr M, Lutz B. The endogenous cannabinoid system protects against colonic inflammation. J Clin Invest. 2004 Apr;113(8):1202-9.

120 Wallace JL, Flannigan KL, McKnight W, Wang L, Ferraz JG, Tuitt D. Pro-resolution, protective and anti-nociceptive effects of a cannabis extract in the rat gastrointestinal tract. J Physiol Pharmacol. 2013 Apr;64(2):167-75. PubMed PMID: 23756391.

121 Singh UP, Singh NP, Singh B, Price RL, Nagarkatti M, Nagarkatti PS. Cannabinoid receptor-2 (CB2) agonist ameliorates colitis in IL-10(-/-) mice by attenuating the activation of T cells and promoting their apoptosis. Toxicol Appl Pharmacol. 2012 Jan 15;258(2):256-67. doi: 10.1016/j.taap.2011.11.005.

122 Coskun ZM, Bolkent S. Oxidative stress and cannabinoid receptor expression in type-2 diabetic rat pancreas following treatment with Δ^9-THC. Cell Biochem Funct. 2014 Oct;32(7):612-9. doi: 10.1002/cbf.3058. Epub 2014 Sep 3.

123 Horváth B, Mukhopadhyay P, Haskó G, Pacher P. The endocannabinoid system and plant-derived cannabinoids in diabetes and diabetic complications. Am J Pathol. 2012 Feb;180(2):432-42. doi: 10.1016/j.ajpath.2011.11.003. Epub 2011 Dec 5. Review.

124 Penner et al. 2013. Marijuana use on glucose, insulin, and insulin resistance among US adults. American Journal of Medicine 126: 583-589.

125 Rajavashisth et al. 2012. Decreased prevalence of diabetes in marijuana users. BMJ Open 2.

126 Alshaarawy O, Anthony JC. Brief Report: Cannabis Smoking and Diabetes Mellitus: Results from Meta-analysis with Eight Independent Replication Samples. Epidemiology. 2015 Jul;26(4):597-600. doi: 10.1097/EDE.0000000000000314.

127 LeStrat Y, LeFoll B. Obesity and Cannabis Use: Results From 2 Representative National Surveys. Am. J. Epidemiol. First published online Aug. 24, 2011. doi:10.1093/aje/kwr200

128 Wallace MS, Marcotte TD, Umlauf A, Gouaux B, Atkinson JH. Efficacy of Inhaled Cannabis on Painful Diabetic Neuropathy. J Pain. 2015 Jul;16(7):616-27. doi: 10.1016/j.jpain.2015.03.008.

129 Hoggart B, Ratcliffe S, Ehler E, Simpson KH, Hovorka J, Lejčko J, Taylor L, Lauder H, Serpell M. A multicentre, open-label, follow-on study to assess the long-term maintenance of effect, tolerance and safety of THC/CBD oromucosal spray in the management of neuropathic pain. J Neurol. 2015 Jan;262(1):27-40. doi: 10.1007/s00415-014-7502-9.

130 Sagredo, et al. 2011. Neuroprotective effects of phytocannabinoid-based medicines in experimental models of Huntington's disease. Journal of Neuroscience Research 89: 1509-1518.

131 Sagredo O, Pazos MR, Satta V, Ramos JA, Pertwee RG, Fernández-Ruiz J. Neuroprotective effects of phytocannabinoid-based medicines in experimental models of Huntington's disease. J Neurosci Res. 2011 Sep;89(9):1509-18. doi: 10.1002/jnr.22682.

132 Laprairie RB, Kelly ME, Denovan-Wright EM. Cannabinoids increase type 1 cannabinoid receptor expression in a cell culture model of striatal neurons: implications for Huntington's disease. Neuropharmacology. 2013 Sep;72:47-57.

133 Valdeolivas S, Satta V, Pertwee RG, Fernández-Ruiz J, Sagredo O. Sativex-like combination of phytocannabinoids is neuroprotective in malonate-lesioned rats, an inflammatory model of Huntington's disease: role of CB1 and CB2 receptors. ACS Chem Neurosci. 2012 May 16;3(5):400-6. doi: 10.1021/cn200114w.

134 Sieradzan, KA, Fox SH, Hill M, Dick JP, Crossman AR, Brotchie JM. 2001. Cannabinoids reduce levodopa-induced dyskinesia in Parkinson's disease: A pilot study. Neurol 57(11):2108-11.

135 Zuardi AW, Crippa JA, Hallak JE, Pinto JP, Chagas MH, Rodrigues GG, Dursun SM, Tumas V. Cannabidiol for the treatment of psychosis in Parkinson's disease. J Psychopharmacol. 2009 Nov;23(8):979-83. doi: 10.1177/0269881108096519. Epub 2008. Sep 18. PubMed PMID: 18801821.

136 Chagas MHN, Eckeli AL, Zuardi AW, Pena-Pereira MA, Sobreira-Neto MA, Sobreira ET, Camilo MR, Bergamaschi MM, Schenck CH, Hallak JEC, Tumas V.,

Crippa JAS. 2014. Cannabidiol can improve complex sleep-related behaviours associated with rapid eye movement sleep behaviour disorder in Parkinson's disease patients: a case series. Journal of Clinical Pharmacy and Therapeutics, 39: 564–566. doi: 10.1111/jcpt.12179

137 Chagas MH, Zuardi AW, Tumas V, Pena-Pereira MA, Sobreira ET, Bergamaschi MM, dos Santos AC, Teixeira AL, Hallak JE, Crippa JA. Effects of cannabidiol in the treatment of patients with Parkinson's disease: an exploratory double-blind trial. J Psychopharmacol. 2014 Nov;28(11):1088-98. doi: 10.1177/0269881114550355.

138 Kohli DR, Li Y, Khasabov SG, Gupta P, Kehl LJ, Ericson ME, Nguyen J, Gupta V, Hebbel RP, Simone DA, Gupta K. Pain-related behaviors and neurochemical alterations in mice expressing sickle hemoglobin: modulation by cannabinoids. Blood. 2010 Jul 22;116(3):456-65. doi: 10.1182/blood-2010-01-260372.

139 Howard J, Anie KA, Holdcroft A, Korn S, Davies SC. Cannabis use in sickle cell disease: a questionnaire study. Br J Haematol. 2005 Oct;131(1):123-8.

140 Russo, Ethan. 2004. Clinical endocannabinoid deficiency (CECD): Can this concept explain therapeutic benefits of cannabis in migraine, fibromyalgia, irritable bowel syndrome and other treatment-resistant conditions? Neuroendocrinology Letters 25: 31-39.

141 Schley, et al. 2006. Delta-9-THC based monotherapy in fibromyalgia patients on experimentally induced pain, axon reflex flare, and pain relief. Current Medical Research and Opinion 22: 1269-1276.

142 Fiz, et al. 2011. Cannabis use in patients with fibromyalgia: Effect on symptoms relief and health-related quality of life. PLoS One 6.

143 Hampson, AJ, Grimaldi M, Axelrod J, Wink D. 1998. Cannabidiol and (-)Delta9-tetrahydrocannabinol are neuroprotective antioxidants. Proc Natl Acad Sci USA 95 (14):8268-73.

144 Fishbein-Kaminietsky M, Gafni M, Sarne Y. Ultralow doses of cannabinoid drugs protect the mouse brain from inflammation-induced cognitive damage. J Neurosci Res. 2014 Dec;92(12):1669-77. doi: 10.1002/jnr.23452. Epub 2014 Jul 16. PubMed PMID: 25042014.

145 Werner, Clint. Marijuana - Gateway to Health, 2011, Dachstar Press.

146 Patent # 6630507. http://patft.uspto.gov/.

147 Wilsey B, Marcotte T, Deutsch R, Gouaux B, Sakai S, Donaghe H. Low-dose vaporized cannabis significantly improves neuropathic pain. J Pain. 2013 Feb;14(2):136-48. doi: 10.1016/j.jpain.2012.10.009.

148 Carter GT, Abood ME, Aggarwal SK, Weiss MD. Cannabis and amyotrophic lateral sclerosis: hypothetical and practical applications, and a call for clinical trials. Am J Hosp Palliat Care. 2010 Aug;27(5):347-56. doi: 10.1177/1049909110369531.

149 Giusti GV, Chiarotti M, Passatore M, Gentile V, Fiori A. Muscular dystrophy in mice after chronic subcutaneous treatment with cannabinoids. Forensic Sci. 1977 Sep-Oct;10(2):133-40.

150 Backes. Cannabis Pharmacy, 2014.

151 Strohbeck-Kuehner P, Skopp G, Mattern R. Cannabis improves symptoms of ADHD. Cannabinoids 2008;3(1):1-3.

152 Kurz R, Blaas K. Use of dronabinol (delta-9-THC) in autism: A prospective single-case-study with an early infantile autistic child. Cannabinoids 2010;5(4):4-6 "There are well known alterations of neurotransmitters in autistic people especially in the cerebral cannabinoid receptor system."

153 Qin M, Zeidler Z, Moulton K, Krych L, Xia Z, Smith CB. Endocannabinoid-mediated improvement on a test of aversive memory in a mouse model of fragile X syndrome. Behav Brain Res. 2015 Sep 15;291:164-71. doi: 10.1016/j.bbr.2015.05.003.

154 Földy C, Malenka RC, Südhof TC. Autism-associated neuroligin-3 mutations commonly disrupt tonic endocannabinoid signaling. Neuron. 2013 May 8;78(3):498-509. doi: 10.1016/j.neuron.2013.02.036. Epub 2013 Apr 11.

155 Ramot Y, Sugawara K, Zákány N, Tóth BI, Bíró T, Paus R. A novel control of human keratin expression: cannabinoid receptor 1-mediated signaling down-regulates the expression of keratins K6 and K16 in human keratinocytes in vitro and in situ. PeerJ. 2013 Feb 19;1:e40. doi: 10.7717/peerj.40.

156 Bíró T, Tóth BI, Haskó G, Paus R, Pacher P. The endocannabinoid system of the skin in health and disease: novel perspectives and therapeutic opportunities. Trends Pharmacol Sci. 2009 Aug;30(8):411-20. doi: 10.1016/j.tips.2009.05.004. Epub 2009 Jul 14.

157 Wilkinson JD, Williamson EM. Cannabinoids inhibit human keratinocyte proliferation through a non-CB1/CB2 mechanism and have a potential therapeutic value in the treatment of psoriasis. J Dermatol Sci. 2007 Feb;45(2):87-92.

158 Fowler CJ. Pharmacological properties and therapeutic possibilities for drugs acting upon endocannabinoid receptors. Curr Drug Targets CNS Neurol Disord. 2005 Dec;4(6):685-96. Review. PubMed PMID: 16375686.

159 Namazi MR. Cannabinoids, loratadine and allopurinol as novel additions to the antipsoriatic ammunition. J Eur Acad Dermatol Venereol. 2005 May;19(3):319-22. Review. Erratum in: J Eur Acad Dermatol Venereol. 2005 Jul;19(4):529.

160 Taylor AH, Ang C, Bell SC, Konje JC. The role of the endocannabinoid system in gametogenesis, implantation and early pregnancy. Hum Reprod Update. 2007 Sep-Oct;13(5):501-13. Epub 2007 Jun 21.

161 Ross JS, Shua-Haim JR. Open-label study of dronabinol in the treatment of refractory agitation in Alzheimer's disease: a pilot study. American Society of Consultant Pharmacists' 34th Annual Meeting, Nov. 12-15, 2003.

162 Eubanks LM, Rogers CJ, Beuscher AE, Koob GF, Olson AJ, Dickerson TJ, Janda KD. A molecular link between the active component of marijuana and Alzheimer's disease pathology. Mol Pharm. 2006 Nov-Dec;3(6):773-7.

163 Conant v. Walters, 309 F. 3d 629. Court of Appeals, 9th Circuit 2002.

164 Kilmer, et al. Marijuana Legalization, Oxford University Press, 2012.

165 MacCoun, RJ. 2011. What can we learn from the Dutch cannabis coffeeshop system? Addiction, 106: 1899–1910. doi: 10.1111/j.1360-0443.2011.03572.x

166 Kilmer, et al. Marijuana Legalization. Oxford University Press, 2012, pg. 43.

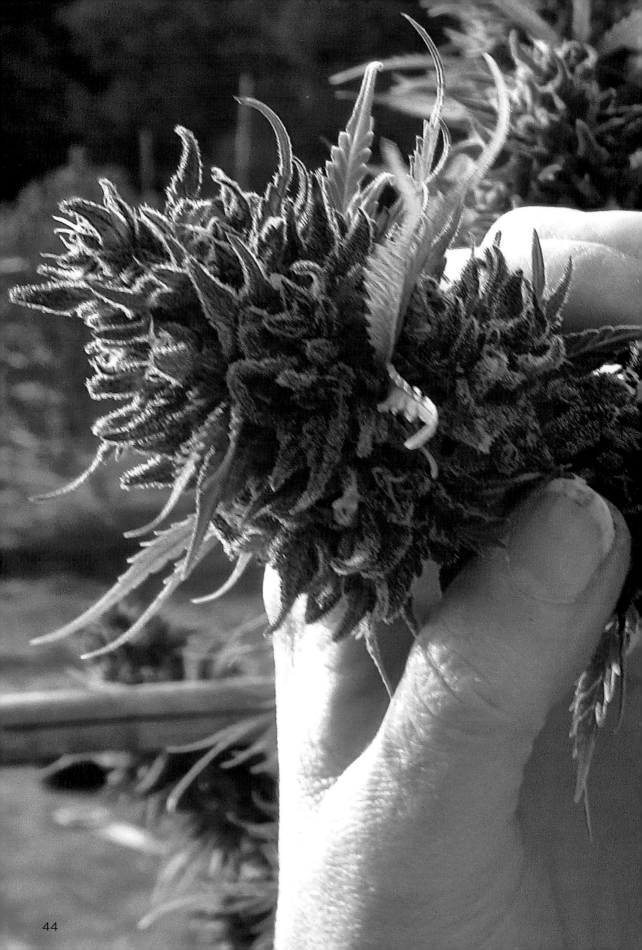

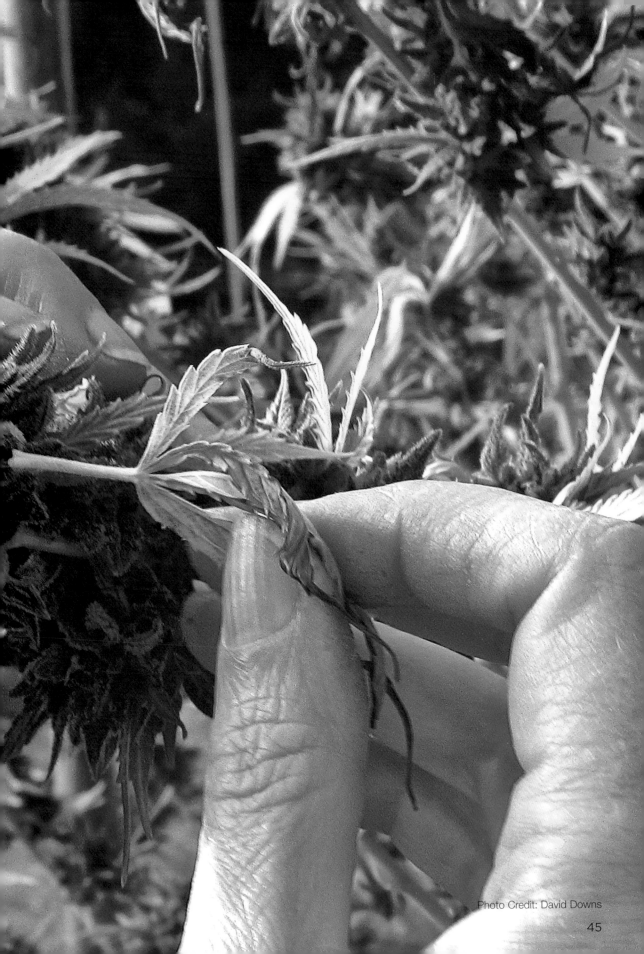

Photo Credit: David Downs

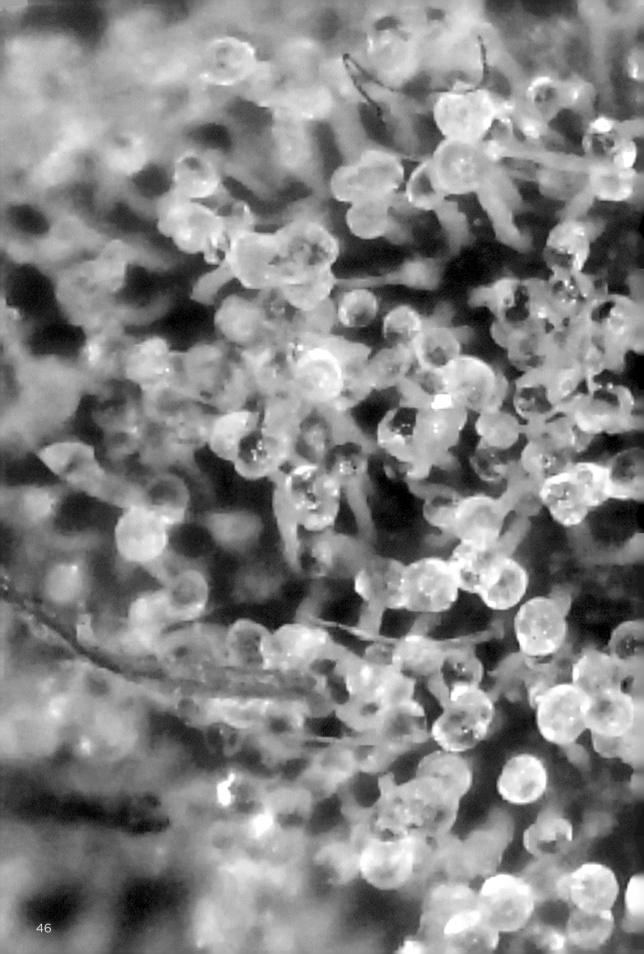

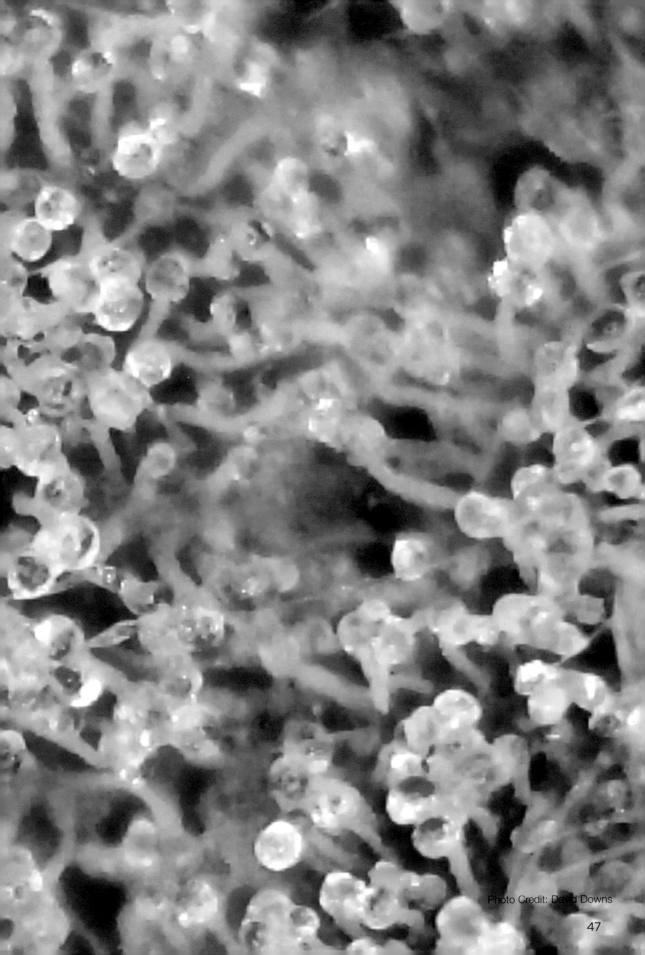

Photo Credit: David Downs

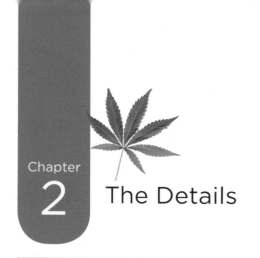

The Details

Medical cannabis has many formulations, from the raw, dried, cured flower buds of the plant to highly processed and refined oils, tinctures and other extracts. Under cannabis prohibition, raw flowers might have been all that was available. But with medical cannabis legalization, producers have the legal freedom to further refine the crop for more specific applications.

Dried Flowers

More Americans have access to dried, cured flower buds of cannabis than probably any other formulation[1]. It's the simplest form of medical cannabis. The plant is grown from a seedling into a bush, then undergoes flowering for about eight weeks. The unfertilized female flower tops are most rich in the plant's medicinal compounds, and at peak ripeness they are cut, dried, trimmed, cured, and stored for later use.

Laws permitting, patients or their caregivers can grow their own supplies of cannabis, or they often purchase them from dispensaries, and collectives.

Cannabis flowers also come in a variety of potencies from low to high, and plants can have widely different levels of their main active ingredients, which we detail later.

Medical cannabis flowers come in two main families: indicas and sativas — now very interbred.

Patients report indicas tend to be more sedative, while sativas are more energetic and less sedative. Indica effects are more sought after for pain relief, insomnia, and muscle tension, while sativa effects are often used for daytime management of anxiety, depression, headaches and bowel diseases. Most cannabis is a hybrid of sativa and indica genetics, but it may have more of one or the other.

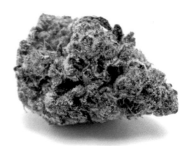

Indica bud.

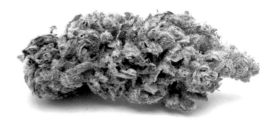

Sativa bud.

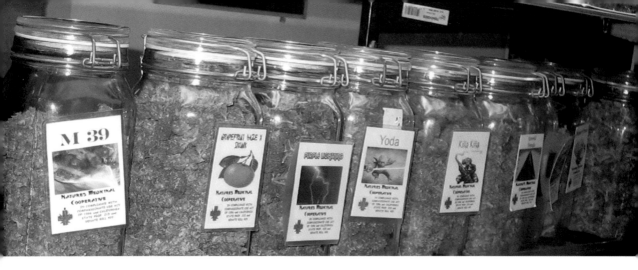

The sativa and indica families come from two different geographical home regions of the plant. Indicas developed in subtropical and temperate climates and at higher altitudes, while sativas come from more tropical regions. The plants not only adapted physically to these different climates, but their effects became different as well.

There are hundreds of different varietals of cannabis — called strains — along the spectrum from a full indica to a full sativa. There is preliminary science to support the very large amounts of patient reports that different cannabis strains can have different effects,[2] probably due to differences in terpene content.

Edibles

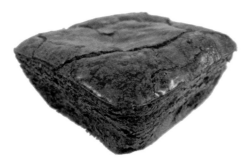

THC-rich brownie.

Next in popularity to flowers on dispensary shelves are edibles, which are foods infused with the active ingredients in cannabis. It can be a brownie, or a cookie, or an entire pepperoni pizza, or a soft drink — you name it.

The active ingredients in cannabis easily transfer into oils or glycerin solutions and are then baked into foods. (The cannabis leaf is filtered out.) Patients are making edibles at home or they are buying them from collectives and dispensaries.

Edibles allow patients to consume cannabis in places where smoking is not allowed, and the effect of edibles can be considerably longer than smoking. Edibles can vary in potency from very weak to extremely strong, and patients should exercise caution and always follow usage instructions.

Extracts

Extracts of cannabis have become as popular or more popular than edibles. The active ingredients in cannabis can be extracted in a variety of different ways for more processed formulations.

Extracts can be multiple times more potent that raw flower buds and can come in a variety of consistencies — from dry-sifted kief to oily and viscous,

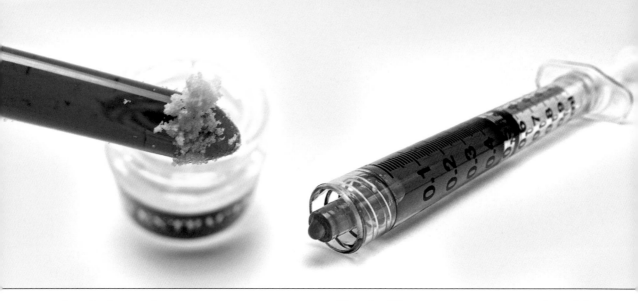

to hard, dry and waxy, or transparent and brittle.[3]

Among the most popular extracts in medical marijuana states is "hash oil." To make cannabis oil, the plant's essential oils and waxes are concentrated through solvent extraction and then purged of the solvent. The most common, cheap and available solvent to make hash oil is butane, but it's flammable, dangerous, and usually illegal. However, extracts made with ice water are very popular, as well as those made with ethyl alcohol or carbon dioxide. Extracts of whole plant botanical cannabis like GW Pharmaceutical's Sativex and Epidiolex are among the most modern and medically accepted formulations available.

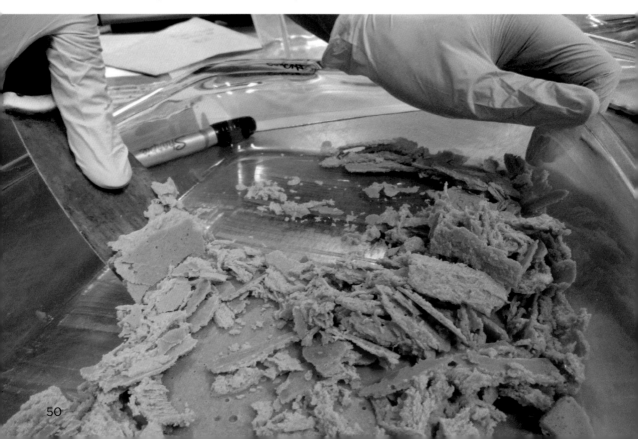

Topicals

An emerging frontier in cannabinoid therapy is the use of balms and ointments infused with the active ingredients in cannabis.

Both the skin and the underlying muscle and nerves contain cell receptors that interact with cannabis' ingredients to decrease inflammation, immune response, act as an anti-bacterial, and potentially as an anti-tumor agent. Cannabis topicals are available in most advanced medical cannabis states, or they can be made at home for relatively cheap using homegrown supplies of cannabis and store-bought coconut oil. Patients also report that infused coconut oil is also effective for female sexual dysfunction and arousal.

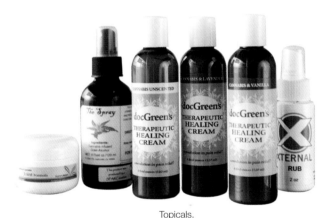

Topicals.

What Is THC?

Prospective medical cannabis patients are going to be hearing a lot about the acronym THC. Simply put, THC is the main active ingredient in cannabis. It's a very small molecule that the plant creates, and THC interacts with a wide variety of cells in the human body to cause many of cannabis' effects, including pain relief, appetite stimulation, and euphoria.

THC (which stands for "delta-9-tetrahydrocannabinol") is one of dozens of active molecules in cannabis called cannabinoids. The plant secretes these compounds for a variety of reasons, including protection from the sun and pests, and reproduction.

For the last 10,000 years, humans have used cannabis as a food, fuel, and fiber, and thanks to THC, as a medicine. Scientists isolated THC in the 1960s, and figured out how it plugged into our cells in the 1990s. Today, the number of indications for THC is vast.

In most modern medical cannabis economies, products are listed with the amount of THC in them the same way alcoholic beverages are listed with the amount of alcohol in them. Medical cannabis flower buds can have anywhere from 1 percent to over 20 percent THC content by dry weight. Extracts can test as high at 99 percent THC. Pure THC can look like a pale, white powder.

What Is CBD?

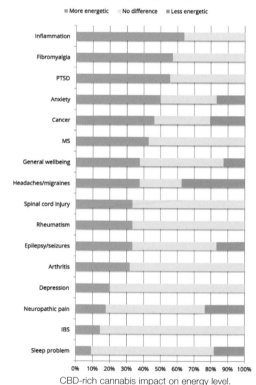
CBD-rich cannabis impact on energy level.

Cannabidiol, or CBD, is the second most common active ingredient in cannabis. It's generally considered non-psychoactive — it doesn't cause euphoria. Patients do report it can make them drowsy.

Cannabidiol has potent anti-inflammatory[4] [5] [6] and immunosupressive properties in cell and animal studies.[7] Research backs up the use of CBD for dozens of indications, including rheumatoid arthritis, types 1 and 2 diabetes, atherosclerosis, Alzheimer disease, hypertension, the metabolic syndrome, ischemia-reperfusion injury, depression, and neuropathic pain.[8] CBD dampens the effects of THC,

and has no psychoactivity of its own[9], and is extremely non-toxic. You can't overdose on CBD. CBD also treats anxiety (though at extremely high doses, patients have reported feeling panicky).[10] CBD may be a future treatment for cancer, and affective and neurodegenerative diseases.

Sixteen states have passed laws that legalize medical uses of CBD, even though CBD remains a federally illegal drug deemed highly addictive and medically useless. The federal government also has a patent on CBD for brain injury during stroke.

In advanced medical cannabis economies, many products list their CBD content in milligrams or as a percentage of the dry weight of the flower. CBD was nearly bred out of black-market cannabis, because it dampens the high of THC. However, with the popularization of CBD, many medical applications and CBD breeding programs have rescued and strengthened CBD-rich plants. Today, dozens of CBD-rich varieties are available in seed and clone in America for use by homegrowing patients, caregivers, collectives and dispensaries.

CBD can also be found in trace amounts in industrial hemp, which is a type of cannabis grown for fiber, seeds, and oil. Efforts are underway to create legal, domestic hemp-based CBD product pipelines.

Combining THC & CBD

More and more patients are learning to use THC and CBD in some form of combination with one another for the best form of relief.

In cases of pediatric epilepsy, caregivers report experimenting with different ratios of CBD:THC, from 1:1 to 20:1, to find what works best to calm seizures. Similarly, arthritis patients will experiment with differing ratios of CBD:THC to find the one that works best for symptom relief.

In nature, THC and CBD co-exist with several dozen other compounds called cannabinoids and aromatic molecules called terpenes that are also therapeutic.

While medical science is mainly focused on single molecules in cannabis that may be effective, there is mounting evidence that cannabinoids work best in concert with one another in what is called The Entourage Effect[11] [12] [13] [14]. Animal studies have found whole-plant CBD works better than CBD alone.[15] Patients regularly report pure, synthetic THC (Marinol, Dronabinol) is less effective on nausea than whole-plant cannabis formulations. And the world's leading medical cannabis pharmaceuticals maker, GW Pharmaceuticals, has pioneered whole-plant extracts in Sativex and Epidiolex.

CBD dampens the euphoria or high of THC, while at the same time lengthening its therapeutic effect. More and more patients are choosing products with low or no THC and a lot of CBD to manage anxiety, pain and inflammation.

> THC, CBD, other cannabinoids and terpenes work together in an entourage ensemble effect.

What is One Dose?

Generally, one dose of medical cannabis is anywhere from 2 to 10 milligrams of THC,[16] depending on a person's size, tolerance, and chemistry. Since CBD is not psychoactive, doses of it can be higher without any noticeable adverse effects (5 to 50 milligrams).

What is a milligram? A milligram is one one-thousandth of a gram, a very small amount.

Let's start with flowers. Dosing varies with medical cannabis flowers due to the variance in the strength of each batch, and the mode of delivery. Flowers can be anywhere from 5 to 23 percent THC and from 0 to 15 percent CBD (with a variance of +/-3 percent). For average-strength flowers (15 percent THC), one starting dose might be a three-second draw on a lit pipe or joint, followed immediately by exhalation.[17] Wait 10 minutes to judge the effect.

For an edible, one dose might be just a sliver of a cookie. Read the edible package for the amount of milligrams in one entire edible item, and figure out what percentage of the edible would be one dose. In Colorado, 10 milligrams is an official state dose of THC. So, a 100mg cookie contains 10 doses, and only one-tenth of a cookie should be consumed every two hours before judging the effect.

Dosing can be very precise with extracts of cannabis in tincture form, which is a potent, swallowable liquid. Depending on the brand, one medicine dropper might equal 5mg of cannabinoids, so read the label. States with medical cannabis testing labs and regulations mandating testing greatly enhance a patient's ability to accurately dose their medicine.

Extracts are more potent than raw cannabis and dosing can be much harder, or easier, depending on the method. Lab testing and labeling for potency work wonders for extracts. Always start with as little extract as medically effective. One great way to dose effectively is with a device like a pen vaporizer. Patients are using oil extracts in pen vaporizers to take tiny sips of cannabis vapor containing a couple milligrams of THC until they achieve the desired level of relief.

How to Safely Use Cannabis
Smoking

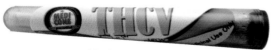
Joint for pain and anxiety.

Patients roll their own joints out of dried cannabis flowers, or purchase joints that are rolled for them. Depending on the strength of the flowers inside, one dose may be a single inhalation off of a lit joint. Onset of effects can be measured in seconds. Do not hold the smoke in. (Most THC transfers rapidly into the blood upon inhalation. Holding smoke in longer results in more irritation.) Resist the impulse to smoke the entire joint so as not to "waste" it. Simply put it out and save it for later.

If you are using a pipe, high-strength borosilicate glass (Pyrex) is best for heat and damage resistance.

A water-filtered pipe (bong, bubbler) cools and filters smoke for a smoother draw. Just keep in mind that you can accidentally take in larger amount of cannabinoids with water filtration, so start with very small draws, then wait 10 minutes, and take more if needed.

Health side note: Occasional and low cumulative marijuana use is not associated with adverse effects on pulmonary function[18]. Longtime cannabis smokers may have a decreased risk of lung cancer compared to non-smokers or tobacco smokers.[19] Chronic smoking can increase risk of bronchitis and respiratory infections.

Tips

Smoking cannabis can cause a sudden drop in blood pressure, so do it sitting down. Wait a minute before getting up, and do so slowly.

When using cannabis, avoid alcohol, lots of sun, and dehydration. All can exacerbate the effects of low blood pressure and lead to fainting.

Keep pipes and bongs clean by washing them individually in a plastic bag containing a couple ounces of 91 percent isopropyl alcohol and rock salt. Agitate until clean, then rinse.

According to the FDA safety sheet for synthetic THC (Marinol), do not drive or operate heavy machinery until you find that you can tolerate THC.

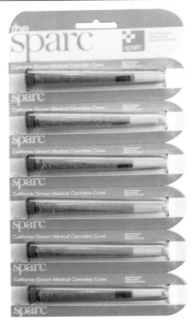

Smokeable medical marijuana.

Vaporizing

Vaporizing is a term encompassing a large class of devices of different sizes that can work with either raw cannabis flowers, or extracts that come in the form of a wax or an oil. Dosage can vary widely with vaporizers.

For vaporizers that take flowers, one dose is roughly equal to what it would be while burning the flowers (one long draw).

For vaporizers that pair with oil extracts, one dose might be a fraction of a draw. Like smoking, the effects of vaporizers come on in seconds, allowing patients to quickly assess their medication levels, and then stop.

Dabbing is the practice of vaporizing and inhaling high-potency cannabis concentrates, usually with a specially designed water pipe. Dabbing can rapidly introduce large amounts of cannabinoids into the blood stream, which is great for certain patients with very severe chronic conditions like multiple sclerosis, but it's also much too strong for the average cannabis patient. Always dab while sitting down.

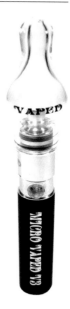

Topical

Rubbing cannabinoids on the skin is a very safe way to use the drug. It also seems to work near instantly, patients have reported[20]. They are using formulations that have a wide band of both active and inactive (acid) versions of cannabinoids like THC, CBD and others.

They are rubbing them on to chronically itching skin, sore joints and muscles as part of massage therapy for local pain and muscle spasm relief without any psychoactive mental effects. The relief from topical cannabinoid therapy lasts for hours. Cannabinoids like CBD and several of cannabis' aromatic oils (called terpenes) may also be used to treat certain types of acne by regulating oil production and killing bacteria.

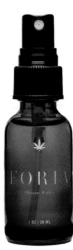

Oral

Some formulations of cannabis are designed to be used in the mouth where they are absorbed through the mucus membranes. Typically these come in the form of lozenges or suckers or cheek strips, and they can be very potent. You have to read the label to determine the amount of milligrams of THC in the product and in one serving of it to figure out what is equal to a starting dose of 2.5 to 5mg. For example, eat one-tenth of a 50mg lollipop (just a sliver) to ingest a 5mg dose of cannabis. Taking medical cannabis this way works slower — under 20 minutes — than smoking or vaping but faster than eating cannabis.

Ingestion

Many formulations of medical cannabis are designed to be eaten, but you need to read the package and label to determine total cannabinoids in the product and what is equal to one dose. Edibles can take anywhere from a half-hour to two hours before onset of effects, and the onset depends on your last meal, size, weight, metabolism, and tolerance. Eaten cannabis' effects can last up to six hours.

For example, if you have a 100mg cookie, cut off one-tenth of it for a 10mg dose and eat just that fraction. Put away the rest for later.

Overdosing on Edibles

Edibles overdoses are common. Commercial edibles are usually potent, and one serving size is often a fraction of a cookie or a brownie. Effects are stronger and can be different than inhaled THC, and can take hours to kick in, which causes patients to eat more than they should.

Always stick to recommended guidelines for edibles and put away uneaten product to avoid accidental ingestion. Read and follow the label's instructions on dosing. Do not consume unlabeled, untested edibles. If you are making your own edibles at home, follow established recipes[21] and opt to include less cannabis rather than more. Eat a very small amount of the product and wait two hours to test the effects.

Over-consuming THC and other cannabinoids can feel disorienting, and nauseating, but it is relatively medically benign. There is no lethal overdose for eaten cannabinoids, but, like any other drug, intoxicated people have hurt or killed themselves or others in accidents. Don't drive on high doses of edibles.

Since anyone can become medicated by an edible, it's also very important to lock them up and keep them away from children, pets, and other adults. Accidental exposure to cannabis can be scary — the person may become tired, confused, dizzy, nauseous and anxious — but it is relatively medically benign. Panicky users who report to the ER usually need no medical treatment. No humans have lethally overdosed on cannabis.[22] Antidotes to THC over-exposure include lemon, pine nuts, and black pepper.[23] The over-the-counter nutraceutical citicholine is another reported antidote to THC intoxication.[24] CBD also dampens THC's effects.

Common-Use Cases

While there are immense research roadblocks to studying which strains are best for which ailment, millions of Americans are conducting what amounts to their own large-scale, uncontrolled clinical trial of different varieties of cannabis for different ailments. In addition to limited human clinical trials, there are vast amounts of patient reports on cannabis' popular indications and modalities of use. A number of groups have online reporting programs[25] to help patients gauge strain effect, and breeders themselves provide reports on effects. More such self-reporting systems are becoming available every day.

Pain[26]

Patients are treating the most common indication for cannabis — pain — in a variety of ways depending on specific ailment and situation.

By far the most common method is smoked or vaporized cannabis flowers that are rich in THC and CBD. Smoking or vaporizing is fast acting and is easy to titrate to find the best dose to manage chronic pain, neuropathy, back pain, fibromyalgia and other types. For stronger, longer lasting pain relief in the body, patients often use ingested forms of the plant. At night, patients use indicas and indica hybrids, including strains with Afghani and Kush genetics for pain relief and sleep. During the day, pain patients report relying on sativa hybrids like Jack Herer, AK-47 and Green Crack. Pain patients often do not want psychoactivity, so high-CBD, low-THC formulations (Harlequin, Sour Tsunami, Harle-Tsu) are often recommended. Cannabinoids do not work as effectively on acute pain.[27]

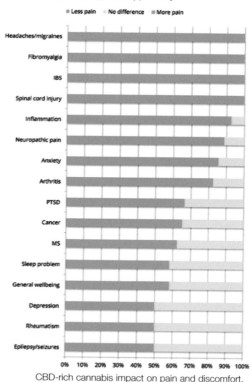

CBD-rich cannabis impact on pain and discomfort.

Note: the colorful strain nomenclature of cannabis reflects its recent roots among popular culture, as opposed to mainstream medicine. In research facilities, new strains generally don't have names, just numbers.

Headaches/Migraine

Cannabis has been used for over 1,000 years to treat headache and migraine, and in modern times, patients are using the botanical in a variety of ways.

Most commonly, raw-plant cannabis or an extract is smoked or vaporized at the beginning of migraine onset to halt migraine progression. Patients also take low-dose prophylactic amounts of THC, like half of a 5mg mint or lozenge to decrease incidence of migraine. Energetic sativas like Super Silver Haze and sativa hybrids like Blue Dream can provide prophylactic effects during the day without fatigue, while more sedative indica hybrids (Cookies, OG Kush) are more appropriate for acute pain and nausea.[28]

Arthritis

Arthritis patients report gravitating toward edible forms of medical cannabis, which do not require smoking and have longer body-centered effects.

They eat indica-dominant edibles (5 to 50mg THC) to reduce pain and sleep through the night. During the day, small smoked or vaporized mixes of combinations of THC and CBD from sativa hybrids like Jack Herer and a CBD-rich variety like Harlequin can help manage pain and inflammation without too much sedation or psychoactivity.

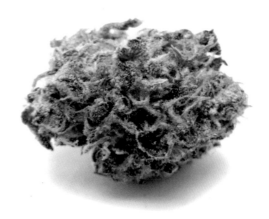

Stress/Anxiety

High doses of THC can cause anxiety, but micro-doses of THC, as well as regular-sized doses of CBD, can lower anxiety. High-CBD flowers (Cannatonic, CBD OG, AC DC, Omrita Rx) are often smoked by people looking to manage stress and anxiety without the high of THC.

Many patients use medical cannabis for stress, and often prefer indica-dominant hybrids like OG Kush and other Kushes to reduce their sense of life's pressures. During the day, low doses of middle-of-the road hybrids like Blue Dream can reportedly decrease anxiety without causing too much psychoactivity.

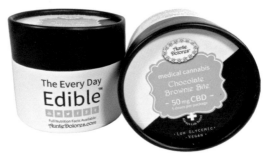

High-CBD brownie for anxiety.

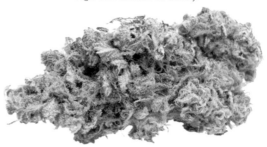

Blue Dream for anxiety.

Nausea, Vomiting, Appetite

Patients report relief from nausea and vomiting using a wide variety of cannabis strains and formulations.

For fast-acting nausea relief, they're using vape pens with hybrid or sativa oil during the day and indicas at night. Smoked flowers work just as well. Oral formulations take longer to begin effects, and might be tough to swallow or keep down. Lozenges, mints and other buccal formulations are almost as fast acting as smoking or vaping.

For appetite, THC-rich indicas often bring on the munchies. By contrast, avoid sativas rich in THC-V — a molecule that suppresses appetite.

Insomnia, Sleep Disorders

Pure indica and indica-dominant flowers are being smoked or vaporized an hour before bedtime for insomnia relief, patients report. For longer-term effects, pure indica and indica-dominant-based edibles are eaten.

Take care to use as low a dose as medically effective. Higher doses of cannabinoids will initially interfere with falling asleep. Popular sleep-aid strains include Aghani, Master Kush, Romulan, Blueberry, and OG Kush. Either high-THC or high-CBD strains can promote sleep, and the effective ratio of THC to CBD can vary widely by patient.

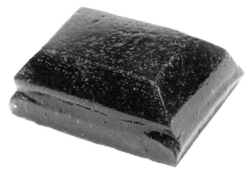

Infused hard candy for sleep.

Cancer

One dose of smoked or vaporized cannabis can be enough to quell the nausea and vomiting of chemotherapy, patients report. One regular dose of inhaled or eaten whole-plant THC and CBD is used to bring on appetite, reduce pain and anxiety, and lift mood.

Patients are also experimenting with highly concentrated extracts of cannabis (greater than 50 percent THC, CBD) topically as an adjunct therapy for pre-cancerous skin lesions, as well as ingesting ultra-high doses of cannabinoids (100s of MGs per day) as an adjunct therapy for brain, breast and colon cancers, among others. No controlled studies of such treatments exist.

Depression

A common and controversial use of medical cannabis, patients report smoking and vaping flowers and extracts of sativa and sativa-hybrid strains (Strawberry Cough, Lemon Thai, etc.) in low doses to manage chronic daytime depression. At night, indica edibles can support sleep and limit insomnia, which reduces depression, patients report.

Gastro-Intestinal

Patients turn to high-THC strains of flowers and their extracts for fast-acting management of the pain, cramping, nausea, and inflammation of Crohn's disease, IBS and other G-I disorders. Smoking or vaping strains like the indicas Afghani and Kush reportedly calms irritated bowels and Crohn's disease, but high-THC sativas work as well.

Why Does Cannabis Have So Many Indications?

Since the beginning of the legalization of medical marijuana, critics have highlighted the number of indications for medical cannabis use that patients have reported. "How can any one plant treat so many things?" became a common critique.

Today, we know why. Over the last 30 years, researchers have figured out that the active ingredients in cannabis plug into a major cell signaling system in the body — like keys into a set of locks.

THC, CBD and dozens of other cannabinoids as well as the aromatic molecules (terpenes) can interact with cell receptors all over the body. These receptors are concentrated in the brain, but they are also found in heavy concentrations in the stomach, in the skin, and throughout the body in immune system cells.

This cell signaling system (the endocannabinoid system) regulates many extremely important activities in the body, including sleep, appetite, sex, immune function, inflammation, and even bone growth.

Researchers are beginning to conclude that dysfunction in the endocannabinoid system might be responsible for a broad array of conditions and diseases.[29]

Cannabinoids interact with this system across all its parameters, which is why the effects of canna-

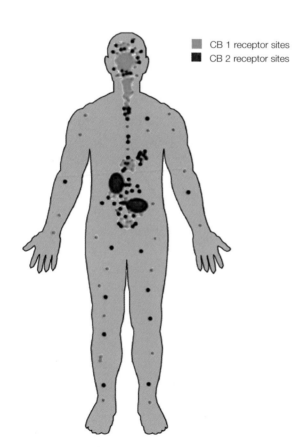

CB 1 receptor sites
CB 2 receptor sites

bis can be so variable and broadly applied. Cannabis contains hundreds of components that can vary by strain and batch, and these components interact with each other in the body, presenting enormous complexity to researchers.

While cannabis and its effects are complex, they're broadly seen as promoting homeostasis — that is, facilitating the body's return to a healthy state of equilibrium.[30] Many symptoms and diseases are caused and exacerbated by a loss of homeostasis, which also partially explains why cannabis is so versatile.

Despite its discovery in the 1990s, the endocannabinoid system is not taught in medical schools. Doctors have little knowledge of this profoundly important system, and how its dysfunction can cause disease and symptoms.

Counter-Indications for Cannabis Use

Cannabis is not a silver bullet for any disease or symptom. Like every drug, it has groups of people for whom it is not considered appropriate.[31]

Pregnancy

Mainstream obstetricians advise against cannabis use before or during pregnancy[32], but the picture is far more complicated.

Cell research shows the endocannabinoid system is involved in regulating all aspects of reproduction, and is probably best left undisturbed by medical cannabis. Smoking cannabis creates the same byproducts and carcinogens as tobacco smoking, which is a known risk factor for pregnant women.

Cannabinoids could interfere with fertility, or actually treat female infertility that is related to [33] certain deficiencies in the female reproductive system. Patients have self-reported using cannabis to treat chronic infertility.

Commonly available drugs for the sometimes intense nausea and vomiting during pregnancy also have side effects, and cannabis may prove a safer option, especially for short, episodic uses.[34] Most studies show no effect of some cannabis exposure on infant mortality.[35]

Children

Generally speaking, giving cannabis-based products to kids is not something doctors recommend. But when it comes to catastrophic, terminal and chronic diseases and conditions that are not responding to conventional therapies, cannabis is increasingly becoming an option[36]. Its side effects are often far more tolerable than conventional pediatric medications for chronic, intractable seizure and/or autism, and cancer symptom management. Pediatricians treating kids with cannabinoids try to avoid smoked formulations in favor of edible oils and tinctures.

Heart Disease

Cannabinoids like THC can increase heart rate and either increase or decrease blood pressure, which raises the risk of heart attack, researchers suspect. This elevated risk could be comparable to the risks from physical activity like running or sex.

Mental Illness

The picture of cannabis use for mental disorders is fuzzy. Conventional medicine warns that someone with a propensity for schizophrenia or psychosis can suffer a quicker onset of the disease with intense cannabis use. THC at high doses can bring on short-term psychosis-like symptoms in some patients. (But so can caffeine and alcohol.)

The intensity of a cannabis experience can cause a psychotic break in people with a predilection to the disease. But other life experiences — moving to college, or losing your virginity — can also precipitate psychotic breaks in people with the tendency.

Conversely, long-term increases in use of cannabis by Americans have not resulted in increases of schizophrenia rates.

And, preliminary data[37] and small trials of CBD for schizophrenia have shown a significant reduction in psychotic symptoms, with fewer side effects than conventional medications.[38][39] Cannabinoids can treat certain metabolic aspects of schizophrenia. Many patients with mental illness are also self-medicating with cannabis.

Bottom line: certain formulations of medical cannabis are helping some people with mental illness, but the wrong formulations of the drug can hurt.

What is Tolerance?

Patients who are prescribed pure, synthetic FDA-approved THC (Dronabinol) are advised to avoid driving "until the drug is tolerated." That's because patients report learning to adapt to and ignore the side effects of cannabis, thus enabling them to function normally.[40][41]

This effect is called tolerance.[42] Your body adjusts to whatever level of THC and CBD it is getting, so that you experience fewer subjective effects of the drug over time. Most patients find their preferred THC level and do not progress into higher levels.[43]

Patients with more severe conditions like cancer and spinal cord injury will often need higher doses of cannabinoids than standard patients, and they also report being able to build up a tolerance to the effects of high doses.

Patients can be taken to very high levels of cannabinoid tolerance without adverse effects.[44] Discontinuing cannabis use brings tolerance quickly back down to a baseline level.

Can You Get Addicted?

Cannabis is less addictive than competing drugs[45], with mild and medically benign withdrawal effects.[46] About 9 percent[47] of people who use cannabis will at one point in their life meet the clinical criteria for dependence.

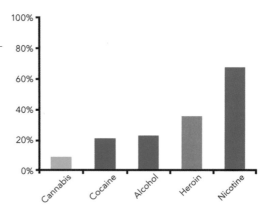

Lifetime probabilities of drug dependence.

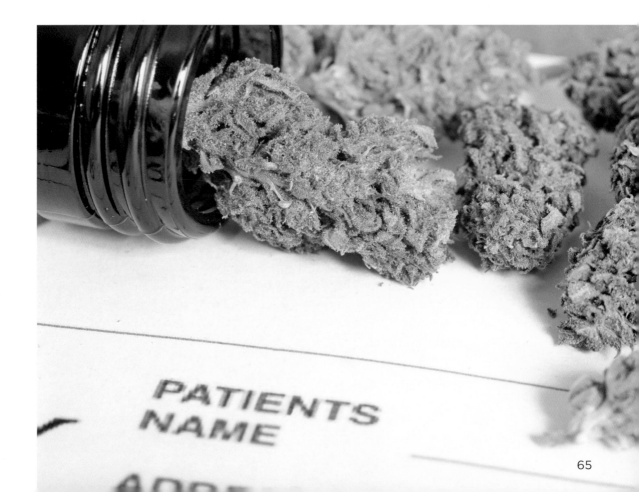

However, the criteria for meeting the definition of dependence includes consequences of use that are not related to health or behavior, but rather societal consequences of prohibition (job loss, expulsion from school). So, the dependence metric of 9 percent is likely too high.[48]

After heavy use, cannabis' physical withdrawal symptoms can include mild insomnia, irritability, reduced appetite, anxiety, and mild depression. Symptoms are easily managed, and usually subside in a few days to two weeks. The body's endocannabinoid system fully returns to its pre-drug state within 28 days.

While physical withdrawal is mild, some people can have a psychological dependence on marijuana, and counseling has proven effective for their underlying issues.

Common Side Effects[49] [50]

Cannabis is one of the safest drugs on the planet, but it can have temporary side effects. Every strain is not right for every patient. Some patients cannot tolerate THC well at all.

Most adverse events are not serious, and dizziness is the most common one[51]. Temporary side effects can include dry mouth, appetite, euphoria, anxiety, low blood pressure, increased heart rate, drowsiness, headache (especially common with too high a dose of THC), forgetfulness, and heightened senses (lights brighter, sounds more audible and detailed)[52]. Onset of negative side effects can help prevent overuse, and they subside in as little as 90 minutes.

Rare side effects — usually involving heavy use — can include feelings of nausea, paranoia, extreme anxiety, dysphoria, allergic reaction, derealization-depersonalization, psychotic break, and hyper-emesis syndrome. They subside with lower doses or discontinued use.

Cannabis' side effects are also a lot safer than common over-the-counter drugs like aspirin and Tylenol, and vastly safer than dangerous painkillers like Vicodin and Oxycontin. And you can't fatally overdose on marijuana.[53]

At high doses, cannabis can cause some people to lose touch with reality, but the same effect can be said for caffeine[54], alcohol, or cough medicine. Always compare the side effects of cannabis against competing drugs when determining safety.

Common Potential Drug Interactions[55][56]

Alcohol
Avoid excess drinking of alcohol with medical cannabis, as they can increase the effects of each other and lead to dizziness, nausea, and vomiting.

Antihistamines
Cannabis can interact with antihistamines to increase heart rate and blood pressure.

Tricyclic Antidepressants
Cannabis can interact with tricyclic antidepressants to increase heart rate and blood pressure.

Amphetamines/Cocaine Other Stimulants
Cannabis can interact with stimulants to increase heart rate and blood pressure.

Opioids
Cannabis can have a positive, synergistic interaction with opioids, allowing patients to use less opioids for the same level of pain relief.

Theophylline
An asthma medication. Using cannabis may decrease theophylline levels in the blood.

Disulfiram or Fluoxetine
A psychiatric drug that may interact with cannabis to cause mild manic episodes, especially in those who are bipolar.

Review of Key Terms

Cannabis
The botanical name for a bushy, cane-like plant with drug properties from Asia that's been used by humans for about 10,000 years as a food, fuel, fiber and medicine.

Marijuana
Mexican folk name for cannabis leaves rolled in cigarette form, beginning in the 1800s. Marijuana became an American legal term for cannabis during the drug's prohibition in the early 1900s, and remains so to this day.

Indica
One of two classifications of medical cannabis. Indicas are said to be more sedative and more often sought out for pain relief. They grow short, fast and stout, and have wide leaves with darker coloring.

Sativa
The second of two families of medical cannabis. Sativas are considered more energetic and with stronger head effects and are used more during the day. Sativas grow tall, slow and thin, with thin leaves.

Hybrid

Hybrids have a mix of indica and sativa genetics, and can be more balanced and versatile than pure sativas or indicas. Hybridized plants also grow easier. In practice, most medical cannabis is heavily hybridized.

Strain

A strain is a particular varietal of cannabis like OG Kush, Blue Dream or Grand Daddy Purple. There are hundreds of different strains, each with slightly different genetics leading to slightly different appearance, feel, smell, taste and effects.[57]

Edibles

Food products infused with the active ingredients in cannabis. Can be difficult to determine proper dosage.

Extracts

Concentrated forms of cannabis that can be multiple times more potent than raw flowers.

Recommendation

The signed, dated document from a doctor qualifying you for medical cannabis.

ID Card

The official state-issued registration identification card — optional or mandatory, depending on which state.

Dispensary

A store that sells medical cannabis products to qualified patients.

Caregiver

A person who is legally allowed to help a patient obtain, grow and or use medical marijuana.

Collective

A group of patients and cultivators who associate to grow and distribute cannabis amongst themselves. A less public, more non-profit entity for medical cannabis distribution.

THC

The main active ingredient in cannabis. THC stands for tetrahydrocannabinol and it is a very small molecule — as opposed to a very large biologic drug — that interacts with the human nervous system to cause cannabis' effects. A product's THC is usually listed in a percentage of dry weight of the flower, or in milligrams in an edible.

CBD

The second most common active ingredient in cannabis. CBD stands for cannabidiol, and it is a very small molecule that interacts with the human nervous system to cause some of cannabis' effects. CBD differs from THC in that it does not cause euphoria, but it does cause sedation. CBD is also anti-epileptic, anti-inflammatory, anti-emetic, muscle relaxant, anxiolytic, neuroprotectant and anti-psychotic, and it reduces the high from THC. A product's CBD is usually listed in a percentage of dry weight of the flower, or in milligrams in an edible.

Dose

A dose of cannabis starts at around 2.5 milligrams of THC, or 5 milligrams of CBD. One effective dose can vary by a person's weight, tolerance and body chemistry. Large, heavy users with a high tolerance can handle 50 mg or 100 mg THC doses. A dose can be equivalent to a small draw off a cannabis cigarette, small puff from a pipe, or a fraction of a marijuana edible.

Milligrams

One thousandth of a gram. A milligram is the scale of measurement used in medical cannabis dosing.

Cannabinoids

The name for the chemicals in the cannabis plant that bind to certain receptors in the body. THC and CBD are the principle cannabinoids, but there are dozens of others in smaller trace amounts found in the plant. Cannabinoids work synergistically to create effects that are more than the sum of their parts.

Terpenes

Terpene is the name for the aromatic molecules in cannabis. Terpenes are responsible for cannabis smell, but they are also therapeutically active and used in combination with the cannabinoids for certain effects like sedation or pain relief. Terpenes can be found throughout the plant kingdom.

Endocannabinoid System

A very important electro-chemical signaling system in human cells, especially nerve cells and immune cells. The system consists of cell receptors (CB1 and CB2) and the molecules that interact with them — the cannabinoids. Your own body makes its own cannabinoids like anandamide, and cannabis is the only plant in nature that also creates cannabinoids.

CB1 Receptor

A primary receptor in the endocannabinoid system and one of the main locations where cannabis creates its effect. CB1 receptors are found in high concentrations in the brain and spine, as well as in the intestines, gonads, and elsewhere. Modulating the CB1 receptor with cannabis can have positive effects on ill people, or it can bring on adverse effects of cannabis in healthy people.

CB2 Receptor

A secondary receptor in the endocannabinoid system, CB2 cells are found mainly in immune cells but also in the brain. Modulating the CB2 receptor with cannabinoids can have positive effects on ill people, or it can bring on adverse effects of cannabis in healthy people.

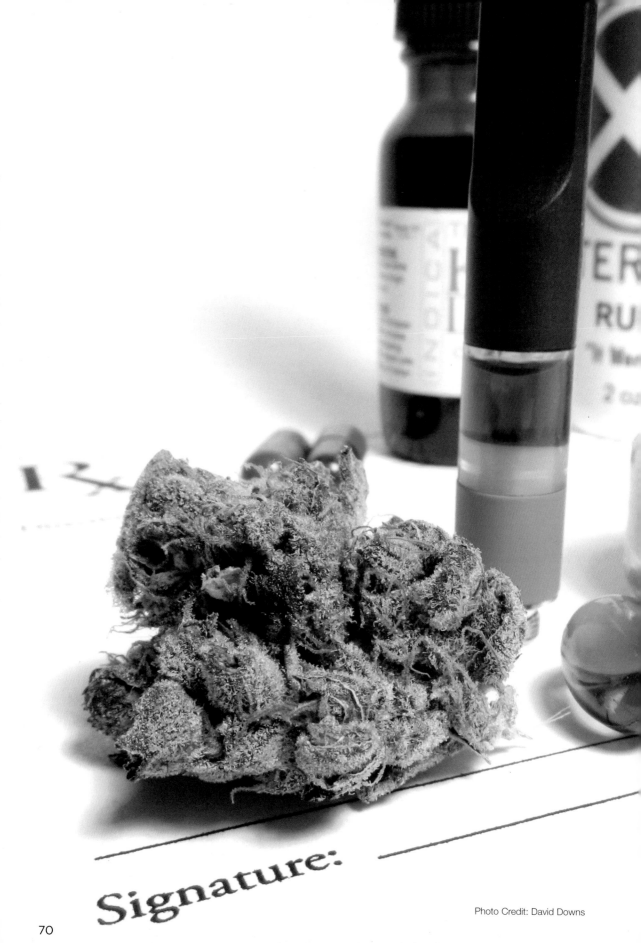

Signature:

Photo Credit: David Downs

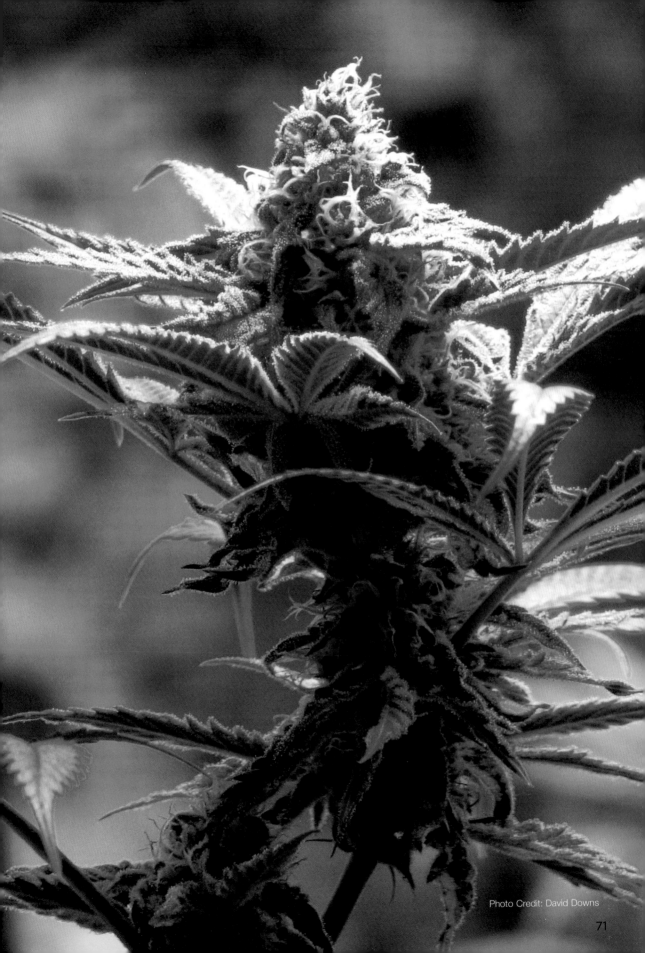

Photo Credit: David Downs

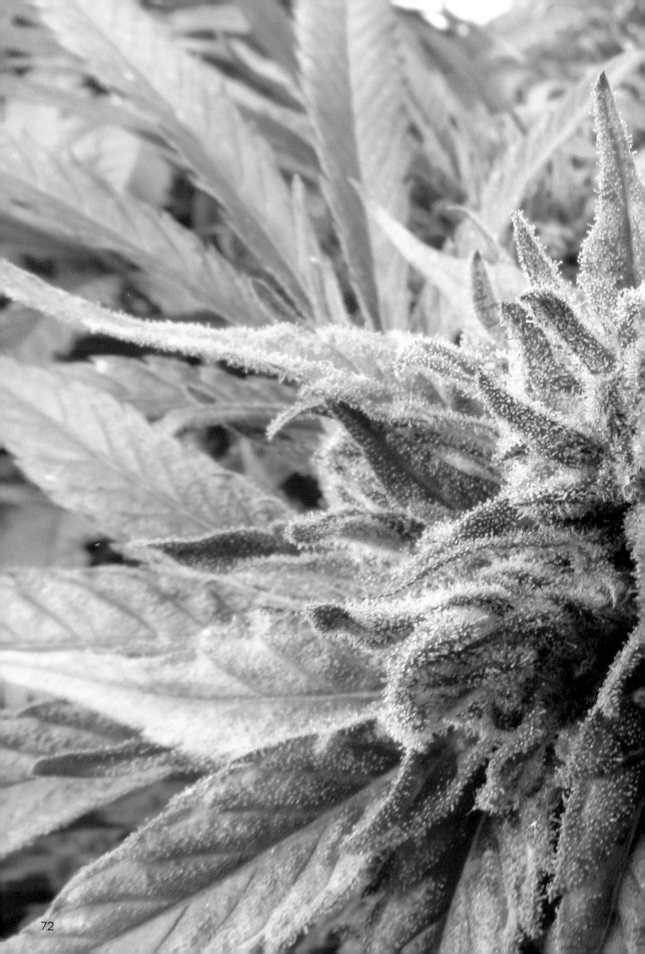

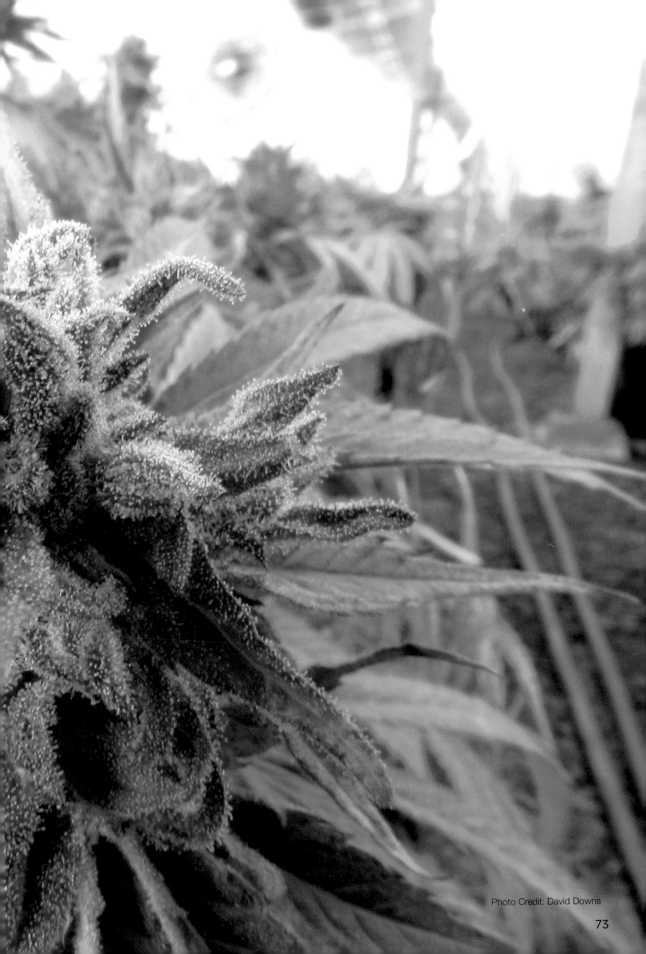

Photo Credit: David Downs

73

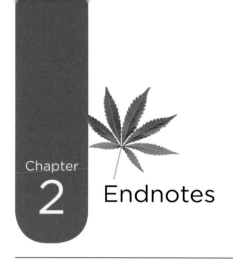

1 UN Drugs Report. 2014.

2 Brunt TM, van Genugten M, Höner-Snoeken K, van de Velde MJ, Niesink RJ. Therapeutic satisfaction and subjective effects of different strains of pharmaceutical-grade cannabis. J Clin Psychopharmacol. 2014 Jun;34(3):344-9. doi: 10.1097/JCP.0000000000000129. PubMed PMID: 24747979.

3 Rosenthal, Ed. Beyond Buds. 2014. Quick Trading.

4 Booz GW. Cannabidiol as an emergent therapeutic strategy for lessening the impact of inflammation on oxidative stress. Free Radic Biol Med. 2011 Sep 1;51(5):1054-61. doi: 10.1016/j.freerad-biomed.2011.01.007.

5 Burstein SH, Zurier RB. Cannabinoids, endocannabinoids, and related analogs in inflammation. AAPS J. 2009 Mar;11(1):109-19. doi: 10.1208/s12248-009-9084-5. Epub 2009 Feb 6. Review.

6 Nagarkatti P, Pandey R, Rieder SA, Hegde VL, Nagarkatti M. Cannabinoids as novel anti-inflammatory drugs. Future medicinal chemistry. 2009;1(7):1333-1349. doi:10.4155/fmc.09.93.

7 Mecha M, Feliú A, Iñigo PM, Mestre L, Carrillo-Salinas FJ, Guaza C. Cannabidiol provides long-lasting protection against the deleterious effects of inflammation in a viral model of multiple sclerosis: a role for A2A receptors. Neurobiol Dis. 2013 Nov;59:141-50. doi: 10.1016/j.nbd.2013.06.016.

8 Booz GW. Cannabidiol as an emergent therapeutic strategy for lessening the impact of inflammation on oxidative stress. Free Radic Biol Med. 2011 Sep 1;51(5):1054-61. doi: 10.1016/j.freerad-biomed.2011.01.007.

9 Dalton WS, Martz R, Lemberger L, Rodda BE, Forney RB. Influence of cannabidiol on delta-9-tetrahydrocannabinol effects. Clin Pharmacol Ther. 1976 Mar;19(3):300-9. PubMed PMID: 770048.

10 Crippa JA, Derenusson GN, Ferrari TB, Wichert-Ana L, Duran FL, Martin-Santos R, Simões MV, Bhattacharyya S, Fusar-Poli P,

Atakan Z, Santos Filho A, Freitas-Ferrari MC, McGuire PK, Zuardi AW, Busatto GF, Hallak JE. Neural basis of anxiolytic effects of cannabidiol (CBD) in generalized social anxiety disorder: a preliminary report. J Psychopharmacol. 2011 Jan;25(1):121-30. doi: 10.1177/0269881110379283. Epub 2010 Sep 9. PubMed PMID: 20829306.

11 Ben-Shabat S, Fride E, Sheskin T, Tamiri T, Rhee MH, Vogel Z, Bisogno T, De Petrocellis L, Di Marzo V, Mechoulam R. An entourage effect: inactive endogenous fatty acid glycerol esters enhance 2-arachidonoyl-glycerol cannabinoid activity. Eur J Pharmacol. 1998 Jul 17;353(1):23-31. PMID:9721036.

12 Russo EB. Taming THC: potential cannabis synergy and phytocannabinoid-terpenoid entourage effects Br J Pharmacol. 2011 Aug;163(7):1344-64. doi: 10.1111/j.1476 5381.2011.01238.x. Review. PMID:21749363.

13 Russo EB. Taming THC: potential cannabis synergy and phytocannabinoid-terpenoid entourage effects. Br J Pharmacol 2011; 163(7): 1344-64.

14 Russo, McPartland. Cannabis and Cannabis Extracts: Greater Than the Sum of Their Parts?; Journal of Cannabis Therapeutics. The Haworth Integrative Healing Press.) Vol. 1, No. 3/4, 2001, pp. 103-132; http://cannabis-med.org/data/pdf/2001-03-04-7.pdf.

15 Gallily R, Yekhtin Z, Hanuš L. 2015. Overcoming the Bell-Shaped Dose-Response of Cannabidiol by Using Cannabis Extract Enriched in Cannabidiol. Pharmacology & Pharmacy, 6, 75-85. doi: 10.4236/pp.2015.62010.

16 Minnesota State Health Dept., http://www.health.state.mn.us/topics/cannabis/practitioners/dosage.pdf.

17 This rule of thumb comports with recent data that estimates .43 grams of marijuana per joint ("What America's Users Spend on Illegal Drugs: 2000-2010," February 2014, White House ONDCP, prepared by Kilmer, et al, RAND Corp) If the flowers were high-quality, and 20 percent THC, then each joint would have 86 milligrams of THC in it. Assuming 10 total draws off the joint, one draw contains 8.6 mgs of THC, of which about half is burned, leaving a 4.6-gram dose for the patient in each inhale.

18 Pletcher MJ, Vittinghoff E, Kalhan R, et al. Association

Between Marijuana Exposure and Pulmonary Function Over 20 Years. JAMA. 2012;307(2):173-181. doi:10.1001/jama.2011.1961.

19 Mehra R, Moore BA, Crothers K, et al.: The association between marijuana smoking and lung cancer: a systematic review. Arch Intern Med 166 (13): 1359-67, 2006.

20 Field reporting, 2009-2015.

21 The Official High Times Cannabis Cookbook. 2012. Elise McDonough.

22 Backes, 2014.

23 Russo EB. Taming THC: potential cannabis synergy and phytocannabinoid-terpenoid entourage effects. Br J Pharmacol. 2011. Aug;163(7):1344-64. doi: 10.1111/j.1476 5381.2011.01238.x. Review.

24 Melamede, interview, 2014.

25 Leafly.com; StickyGuide.com; seedfinder.EU; Big Book of Buds Vol. 1-4. Quick Trading.

26 Russo, EB. 2002. Role of cannabis and cannabinoids in pain management. In Pain management: A practical guide for clinicians, edited by R.S. Weiner. Boca Raton, FL. CRC Press.

27 Backes, 2014.

28 Backes, 2014.

29 Russo.

30 Pertwee.

31 Kahan M, Srivastava A, Spithoff S, Bromley L. Prescribing smoked cannabis for chronic noncancer pain: preliminary recommendations. Can Fam Physician. 2014 Dec;60(12):1083-90. PubMed PMID: 25500598; PubMed Central PMCID: PMC4264803.

32 Marijuana use during pregnancy and lactation. Committee Opinion No. 637. American College of Obstetricians and Gynecologists. Obstet Gynecol 2015;126:234–8.

33 Taylor AH, Ang C, Bell SC, Konje JC. The role of the endocannabinoid system in gametogenesis, implantation and early pregnancy. Hum Reprod Update. 2007 Sep-Oct;13(5):501-13. Epub 2007 Jun 21.b "CB1 receptor deficiencies in some women may have a role to play in tubal pregnancy or female infertility … either inhibited or enhanced cannabinoid signaling impairs embryo transport."

34 Russo, 2003.

35 Fergusson DM, Horwood LJ, Northstone K. Maternal use of cannabis and pregnancy outcome. ALSPAC Study Team. Avon Longitudinal Study of Pregnancy and Childhood. BJOG 2002;109:21–7.

36 Russo, 2003.

37 Robson PJ, Guy GW, Di Marzo V. Cannabinoids and schizophrenia: therapeutic prospects. Curr Pharm Des. 2014;20(13):2194-204. Review. PubMed PMID: 23829368.

38 Leweke FM, Koethe D, Gerth CW, et al. Cannabidiol as an antipsychotic. A double-blind, controlled clinical trial on cannabidiol vs amisulpride in acute schizophrenia. Eur Psychiatry 2007; 22: S14.02.

39 Crippa JA, Zuardi AW, Hallak JE. [Therapeutical use of the cannabinoids in psychiatry]. Rev Bras Psiquiatr. 2010 May;32 Suppl 1:S56-66. Review. Portuguese. PubMed PMID: 20512271.

40 Desrosiers NA, Ramaekers JG, Chauchard E, Gorelick DA, Huestis MA. Smoked cannabis' psychomotor and neurocognitive effects in occasional and frequent smokers. J Anal Toxicol. 2015 May;39(4):251-61. doi: 10.1093/jat/bkv012. Epub 2015 Mar 4. PubMed PMID: 25745105; PubMed Central PMCID: PMC4416120.

41 Theunissen EL, Kauert GF, Toennes SW, Moeller MR, Sambeth A, Blanchard MM, Ramaekers JG. Neurophysiological functioning of occasional and heavy cannabis users during THC intoxication. Psychopharmacology (Berl). 2012 Mar;220(2):341-50. doi: 10.1007/s00213-011-2479-x. PubMed PMID: 21975580; PubMed Central PMCID: PMC3285765.

42 Lichtman AH, Martin BR. Cannabinoid tolerance and dependence Cannabinoids. Handbook of Experimental Pharmacology 2005Springer-Verlag: Heidelberg; 691–717.717In: Pertwee RG (ed). Vol 168.

43 Hoggart B, Ratcliffe S, Ehler E, Simpson KH, Hovorka J, Lejko J, Taylor L, Lauder H, Serpell M. A multicentre, open-label, follow-on study to assess the long-term maintenance of effect, tolerance and safety of THC/CBD oromucosal spray in the management of neuropathic pain. J Neurol. 2015 Jan;262(1):27-40. doi: 10.1007/s00415-014-7502-9. Epub 2014

Sep 30. PubMed PMID: 25270679.

44 Gorelick DA, Goodwin RS, Schwilke E, Schwope DM, Darwin WD, Kelly DL, McMahon RP, Liu F, Ortemann-Renon C, Bonnet D, Huestis MA. Tolerance to effects of high-dose oral 9-tetrahydrocannabinol and plasma cannabinoid concentrations in male daily cannabis smokers. J Anal Toxicol. 2013 Jan-Feb;37(1):11-6. doi: 10.1093/jat/bks081. Epub 2012 Oct 16. PubMed PMID: 23074216; PubMed Central PMCID: PMC3584989.

45 Bostwick JM. Blurred Boundaries: The Therapeutics and Politics of Medical Marijuana. Mayo Clinic Proceedings. 2012;87(2):172-186. doi:10.1016/j.mayocp.2011.10.003.

46 Fox, Armentano, Tvert. Marijuana is Safer: So Why Are We Driving People to Drink? 2013.

47 Catalina Lopez-Quintero, et al. "Probability and Predictors of Transition From First Use to Dependence on Nicotine, Alcohol, Cannabis, and Cocaine: Results of the National Epidemiologic Survey on Alcohol and Related Conditions (NESARC)." Drug and Alcohol Dependence, 2011 May 1; 115(1-2): 120-130. doi:10.1016/j. drugalcdep.2010.11.004

48 Dr. Sunil Aggarwal, 2014.

49 Thompson AE. Medical Marijuana. JAMA. 2015;313(24):2508. doi:10.1001/jama.2015.6676.

50 Whiting PF, Wolff RF, Deshpande S, et al. Cannabinoids for Medical Use: A Systematic Review and Meta-analysis. JAMA. 2015;313(24):2456-2473. doi:10.1001/jama.2015.6358.

51 Tongtong Wang, MSc, Jean-Paul Collet, PhD MD, Stan Shapiro, PhD, and Mark A. Ware, MBBS MSc. Adverse effects of medical cannabinoids: a systematic review CMAJ June 17, 2008. 178:1669-1678; doi:10.1503/cmaj.071178.

52 Arizona Dept of Health Services, http://www.azmedmj.com/side-effects.

53 Sidney S, Beck JE, Tekawa IS, Quesenberry CP, Friedman GD. Marijuana use and mortality. American Journal of Public Health. 1997;87(4):585-590.

54 http://www.healthline.com/health/caffeine-overdose#Overview1

55 Arizona Dept of Health Services, http://www.azmedmj.com/marijuana-other-drugs.

56 FDA, Dronabinol, NDA. 2004, http://www.fda.gov/ohrms/dockets/dockets/05n0479/05N-0479-emc0004-04.pdf.

57 Fischedick JT, Hazekamp A, Erkelens T, Choi YH, Verpoorte R. Metabolic fingerprinting of Cannabis sativa L., cannabinoids and terpenoids for chemotaxonomic and drug standardization purposes. Phytochemistry. 2010 Dec;71(17-18):2058-73. doi:10.1016/j.phytochem.2010.10.001.

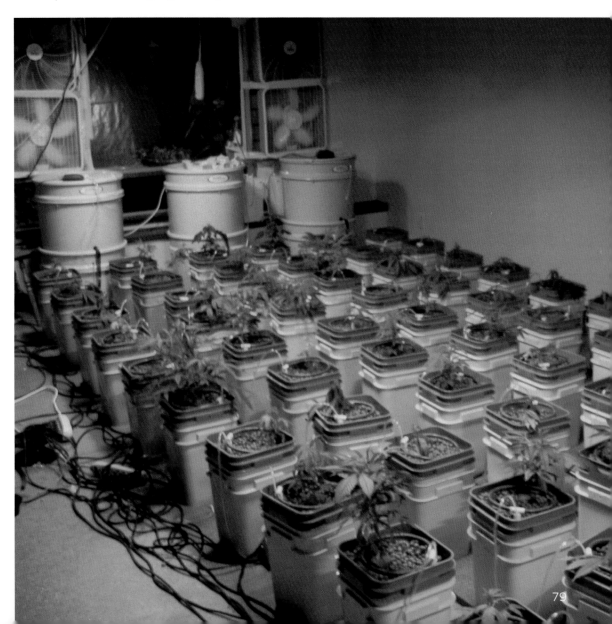

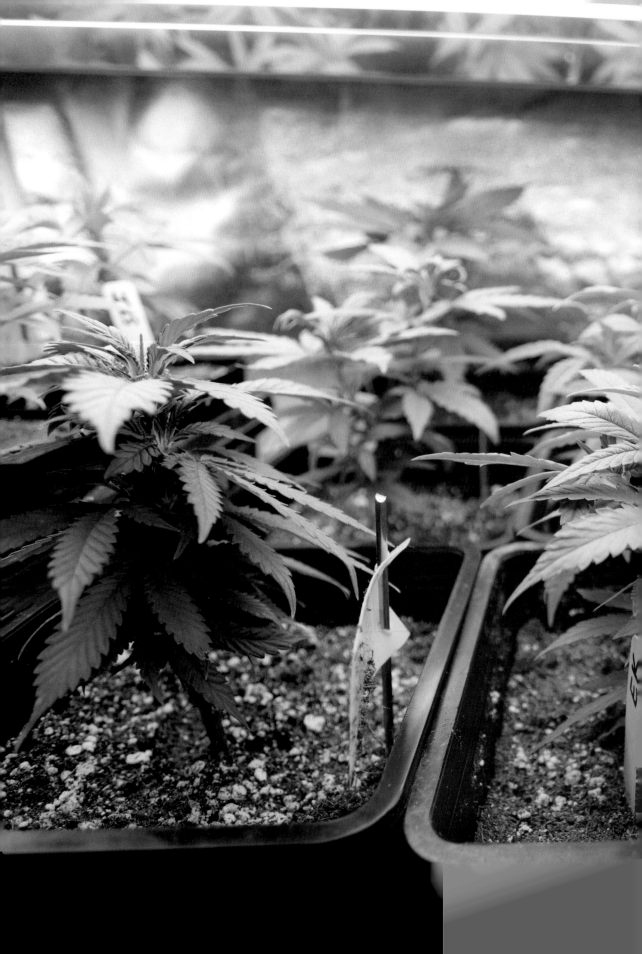

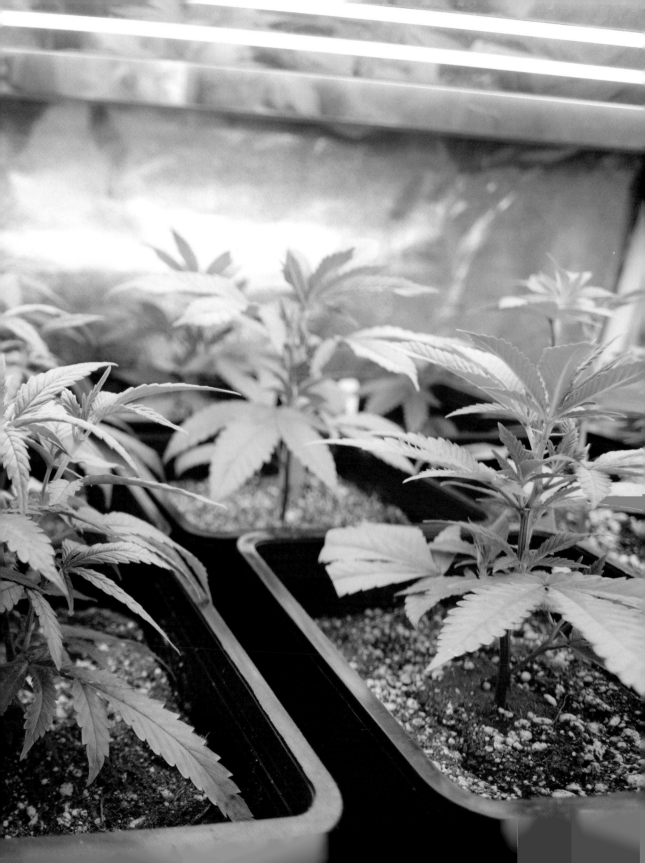

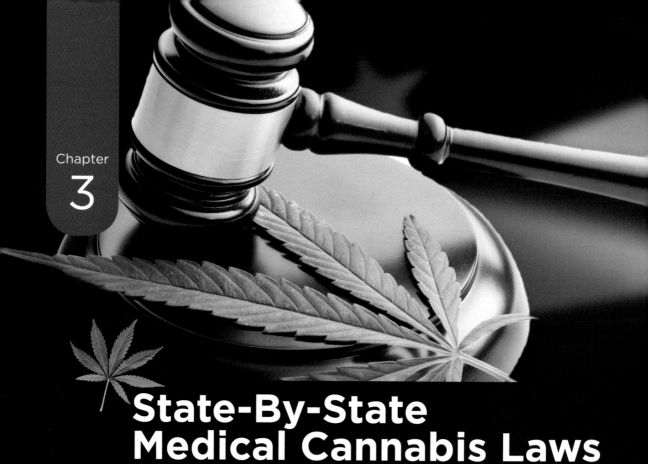

State-By-State Medical Cannabis Laws

The United States has 23 states with medical marijuana laws, 16 states with some form of a CBD law, and 11 states with no legal provisions for medical cannabis whatsoever. Additionally, four states and Washington, D.C., have full adult-use legalization of cannabis, which can hugely benefit those in need.

What follows are the states with medical marijuana laws and how to access their programs, followed by how to access CBD in CBD-states, where possible. For more information on the 11 no-access states and what to do if you live there, see Chapter 4: Resources.

Each state system has similar components, including a medical marijuana law, qualifying conditions, limits, need for a doctor's recommendation, ID card, and outlets like dispensaries.

Wherever possible, we include links in the endnotes to the appropriate application forms to download, complete and submit to become a patient or caregiver in each state.

We also include an overall legal access rating for the state: at the highest is "Easy," followed by "Medium," "Hard" and "Impossible."

Alaska Access Rating: Medium

Recreational Legalization

Alaskans legalized cannabis for recreational use by adults ages 21 and older in 2014 by passing Measure 2. Adults ages 21 and older can legally possess up to one ounce of marijuana, as well as paraphernalia, and grow up to six plants. State-licensed commercial growing facilities and retail stores are slated to open in 2016.

Medical Law

Alaska Measure 8 (passed in 1998) created an affirmative defense against prosecution for certain marijuana crimes.

Qualifying Medical Conditions

Cachexia, cancer, chronic pain, epilepsy and other seizure disorders, glaucoma, HIV or AIDS, multiple sclerosis and other muscle spasticity disorders, and nausea. Other conditions subject to approval by the Alaska Department of Health and Social Services.

Limits

Patients (or their primary caregivers) may legally possess no more than one ounce of usable marijuana, and may cultivate no more than six marijuana plants, of which no more than three may be mature.

Doctor's Recommendation

Physician's recommendation must be based upon a bona fide physician-patient relationship that includes: a review of the patient's medical history and current medical condition; an in-person physical exam; documentation of findings, diagnoses, and recommendations — including a review of other approved medications that may also work.

ID Card

The Alaska Department of Health and Social Services Division of Public Health administers the state's Medical Marijuana Registry Card program, which is confidential. Program enrollment is mandatory in order to have an affirmative medical defense against prosecution for certain marijuana crimes.

The Alaska Bureau of Vital Statistics provides the application for a Registry Card. It costs $25 to apply and you need to fill out the application form available online[1] and include a "Physician Statement." Patients who are minors need written parental consent.

A Physician's Statement must be submitted with the application as the original, signed form — or a certified copy — stating the patient has been

Alaska Access Rating: Medium

diagnosed with a qualifying debilitating medical condition, and the physician concludes the patient might benefit from the medical use of marijuana. The physician must be licensed to practice medicine in Alaska, or an officer in the regular medical service of the armed forces or the United States Public Health Service, or a volunteer without pay to a hospital, clinic or medical office in Alaska.

A photocopy of applicant's Alaska Driver's License or Alaska Identification Card must be included with the application.

Complete the application, and mail it with the physician's statement and check (with pre-printed patient name and address) or money order for $25 (payable to the Bureau of Vital Statistics) to: Alaska Bureau of Vital Statistics, Medical Marijuana Registry, P.O. Box 110699, Juneau, AK 99811-0699.

The renewal application fee is $20. Certain felony convictions or being on probation or parole may disqualify an applicant. Primary and Alternate Caregivers (age 21 and older) may also sign on to the patient's application.

Caregivers
Alaska allows for caregivers and alternate caregivers, via the Registry Card application process explained above.

Medical Dispensaries
Alaska has no lawfully permitted medical marijuana dispensary system, and access is mostly limited to personal medical cultivation, and private medical marijuana patients' association.

---

1 http://dhss.alaska.gov/dph/VitalStats/Documents/PDF.s/MedicalMarijuana.pdf.

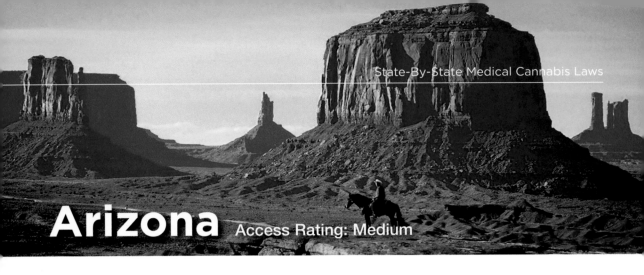

Arizona Access Rating: Medium

Medical Law

The Arizona Medical Marijuana Act (2010) immunizes qualified patients and providers from prosecution for certain marijuana crimes and also prohibits certain discrimination against patients who are students, renters, and employees.

Qualifying Medical Conditions

Alzheimer's disease, amyotrophic lateral sclerosis (Lou Gehrig's disease), cachexia or wasting syndrome, cancer, chronic pain, Crohn's disease, glaucoma, hepatitis C, HIV or AIDS, nausea, persistent muscle spasms, PTSD, seizures.

Limits

Two and half ounces of usable marijuana. Cultivation only allowed if at least 25 miles from nearest licensed dispensary. No more than 12 plants in an "enclosed, locked facility."

Doctor's Recommendation

You have to get a physician to complete a medical records review and an in-person exam, and fill out a Medical Marijuana Physician Certification Form[2]. Cannabis-specialized clinicians are available in Arizona through online directories like WeedMaps.com and Yelp.com.

ID Card

Mandatory. Submit completed online-only application form (available at azdhs.gov[3]), including doctor's certification form, a current passport-style photo (square, between 600 to 1,200 pixels wide), copy of valid identification, signed official Attestation[4] you won't divert marijuana, and valid VISA or MasterCard payment information (credit, debit or prepaid) to cover the $150 initial registration fee. Renewals are $150, and $200 for caregiver. (Application fee reduced to $75 for SNAP/food stamp recipients.) There were 61,153 active patients in Arizona in 2014.

Patients under 18 can join with parent or guardian much the same way as adults, but with a signed and dated "Minor Qualifying Patient New Application" as well as "Medical Marijuana Custodial Parent and Legal Guardian Attestation" form, caregiver picture and fingerprints[5].

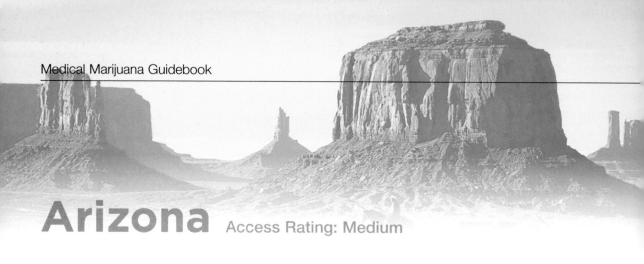

Arizona Access Rating: Medium

Caregivers

Yes, with signed caregiver request form included with patient application, as well as separate Designated Caregiver application. Form includes fingerprinting and FBI criminal background check. Caregivers can have up to five patients. There were 521 active caregivers in Arizona in 2014.

Medical Dispensaries

In 2014 there were 85 state-licensed dispensaries in Arizona. They can be found on Yelp.com, WeedMaps.com, Leafly.com, and other sites.

2 http://azdhs.gov/documents/preparedness/medical-marijuana/physicians/MMJ_PhysicianCertificationForm.pdf.

3 http://azdhs.gov/documents/preparedness/medical-marijuana/patients/adult-patient-application-checklist.pdf.

4 http://azdhs.gov/documents/preparedness/medical-marijuana/patients/Patient_Attestation_Form.pdf.

5 http://azdhs.gov/documents/preparedness/medical-marijuana/patients/patient-under-18-application-checklist.pdf.

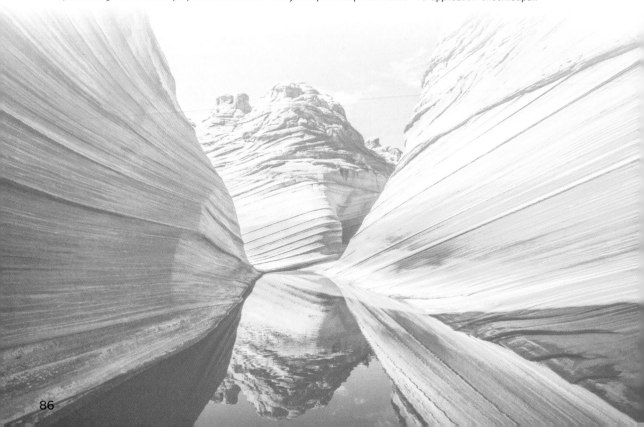

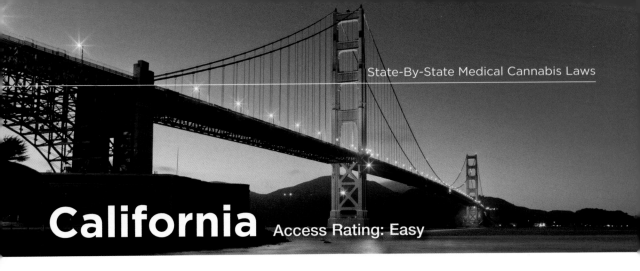

California Access Rating: Easy

Medical Law

Proposition 215, the Compassionate Use Act of 1996, was the nation's first medical marijuana law. It created a limited immunity from prosecution for certain marijuana crimes like possession or cultivation committed by a qualified patient or caregiver. It allows doctors to recommend cannabis. A second law, SB 420, immunized collectives and cooperatives, which laid the groundwork for dispensaries. California passed comprehensive new regulations in 2015 that take effect by 2018. Check www.usmmj.org for complete updates.

Qualifying Medical Conditions

Cancer, anorexia, AIDS, chronic pain, spasticity, glaucoma, arthritis, migraine or "any other illness for which marijuana provides relief."

Limits

Patients are allowed to possess and cultivate as much is reasonably related to their medical need. However, the state's Attorney General's Guidelines specify possessing less than eight ounces of dried marijuana, and growing no more than six mature or 12 immature plants.

Doctor's Recommendation

Patients can get a recommendation for cannabis from a physician licensed by the medical board of California or the Osteopathic Medical Board of California. Most choose to use a cannabis-specialized doctor who focuses exclusively on determining if a person qualifies for medical cannabis. According to the state Attorney General's Guidelines: "A recommending physician is a person who (1) possesses a license in good standing to practice medicine in California; (2) has taken responsibility for some aspect of the medical care, treatment, diagnosis, counseling, or referral of a patient; and (3) has complied with accepted medical standards a reasonable and prudent physician would follow when recommending medical marijuana." Doctors are easy to find in online directories.

ID Card

In 2003, the state legislature passed SB 420 setting up a voluntary confidential medical marijuana patient identification card program. Holders of the state ID are immune from arrest on suspicion of certain marijuana crimes. For the ID, submit a completed application[6] to the county public health

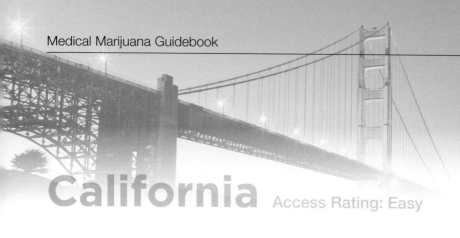

California Access Rating: Easy

department where you reside. Contact your local county health department for office locations, details, and identification card fees. You will need a valid form of photo identification, a proof of residency like utility bills, valid vehicle registration, rent/mortgage receipt, and written recommendation for cannabis from your doctor. Doctors can optionally use a Written Documentation of Patient's Medical Records form (CDPH 9044). Medi-Cal enrollees can get a 50 percent reduction in fees

Caregivers

Primary caregivers are defined under Prop 215 as an "individual designated by the person exempted under this act who has consistently assumed responsibility for the housing, health or safety of that person." It's an option for patients seeking the voluntary state ID to designate a caregiver and apply for their ID card.

Medical Dispensaries

There are several thousand private collectives as well as publicly listed medical cannabis dispensaries. Many cities like San Francisco license and regulate dispensaries, but many others like Fresno ban dispensaries and/or delivery services. The best resources for locating California dispensaries are WeedMaps.com, StickyGuide.com and Leafly.com.

---

6 http://www.cdph.ca.gov/pubsforms/forms/CtrldForms/cdph9042.pdf.

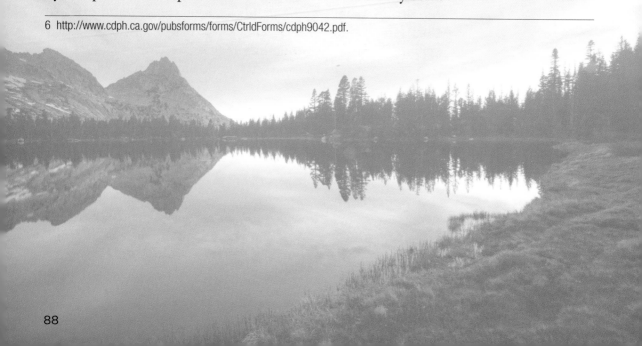

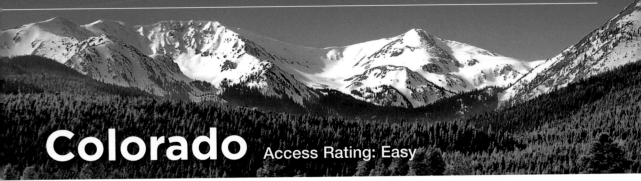

Colorado Access Rating: Easy

Recreational Legalization

Colorado legalized marijuana for adults 21 and over in 2012 and was the first state in the nation to do so. Adults 21 and over can possess up to one ounce of dried marijuana, grow up to six plants (three mature), and buy from hundreds of licensed, taxed and regulated dispensaries.

Medical Law

Colorado legalized medical marijuana in 2000 with Amendment 20. Patients — and their caregivers — with a valid doctor's recommendation to use marijuana have an affirmative defense against prosecution for certain marijuana-related crimes.

Qualifying Conditions

Cancer; glaucoma; HIV/AIDS or treatment for such conditions; a chronic or debilitating disease or medical cachexia; severe pain; severe nausea; seizures, including those that are characteristic of epilepsy; persistent muscle spasms, including those that are characteristic of multiple sclerosis; or any other medical condition, or treatment for such condition, approved by the state health agency. (Denied conditions include asthma, atherosclerosis, bi-polar disease, Crohn's disease, diabetes mellitus types 1 & 2, diabetic retinopathy, hepatitis C, hypertension, Methicillin-Resistant Staphylococcus Aureus (MRSA), opioid dependence, Post Traumatic Stress Disorder (PTSD), severe anxiety and clinical depression, Tourette's syndrome.)

Limits

Up to two ounces dried marijuana and six plants (three mature, three immature).

Doctor's Recommendation

Medical doctors in good standing and licensed to practice medicine in the state of Colorado have protections from prosecution for recommending marijuana, based on an assessment of the patient's medical history, current medical condition and a bona fide physician-patient relationship, and have a copy of their current DEA certificate on file. Cannabis-specialized doctors are widely available in Colorado and can be found through Yelp.com and other online resources.

ID Card

Mandatory. Submit a completed notarized application form[7] to the state department of health, including the original or a copy of written marijuana recommendation, patient and physician's contact information and

Colorado Access Rating: Easy

that of the patient's primary caregiver, if one is designated at the time of application. You need to be a Colorado resident with a valid Social Security Number, and submit a copy of Colorado ID or a complete Proof of Residency Waiver Request form, and the application fee of $15 (payable by check or money order to CDPHE) with your application packet. Applications accepted by mail, physical drop box, or email.[8]

For minors or an authorized representative, include a copy of the guardian's or authorized representative's ID, legal documentation granting legal guardianship or authorized representation including court-certified guardianship documents, power of attorney or medical power of attorney. Medical care rights must be a legally assigned responsibility of the guardian/agent. There are 112,859 active patients in Colorado.

Caregivers

Defined as a person 18 years of age or older who has "significant responsibility for managing the well-being of a patient." Can be added to patient application with a Caregiver Acknowledgement Form. Caregiver registration is mandatory as of May 2015. Limited to five patients and cultivation of 36 plants.[9]

Medical Dispensaries

Thanks to 2010 law, Colorado has hundreds of licensed medical marijuana centers. You can find them on various Internet directories and through advertising, and through the state's Marijuana Enforcement Division.[10]

---

7 https://www.colorado.gov/pacific/sites/default/files/CHED-MMR1001-ADULT-APPLICATION-110114.pdf.

8 https://www.colorado.gov/pacific/cdphe/contact-us-71.

9 https://www.colorado.gov/pacific/sites/default/files/SB15-014.pdf.

10 https://www.colorado.gov/pacific/sites/default/files/Centers%2007012015.pdf.

Connecticut Access Rating: Hard

Medical Law

Medical marijuana has been legal since 2012 under HB 5389, which provides qualified patients and caregivers protection from arrest for certain marijuana crimes.[11]

Qualifying Conditions

Cancer, glaucoma, HIV/AIDS, Parkinson's disease, multiple sclerosis, spinal cord damage with intractable spasticity, epilepsy, cachexia, wasting syndrome, Crohn's disease, Post Traumatic Stress Disorder, sickle cell disease, post laminectomy syndrome with chronic radiculopathy, severe psoriasis and psoriatic arthritis, amyotrophic lateral sclerosis, ulcerative colitis, fabry disease or any medical condition, medical treatment or disease approved by the Department of Consumer Protection.

Limits

A "reasonably necessary" one-month supply of dried cannabis — usually 2.5 ounces. No personal cultivation.

Doctor's Recommendation

You need a written certification by a physician based upon the physician's professional opinion after having completed a medically reasonable exam of the qualifying patient's medical history and current condition made in the course of a bona fide physician-patient relationship. Bring medical records of diagnosis for a qualifying condition. Connecticut has a number of medical cannabis clinics.

ID Card

Mandatory. Your doctor or clinic files your registration[12] for the program and contact information with the Department of Consumer Protection[13]. The DCP will contact you to submit proof of identity, residency, current passport-sized photo, $100 registration fee for you and, if needed, your caregiver. Your physician can indicate to the DCP if you need a caregiver, then you must register the qualified caregiver. Renewals are annual. Connecticut has 4,097 registered patients as of June 2015. Minors allowed with designated guardian and Minor Patient Application.

Caregivers

A primary caregiver must be 18 or older, and can have one qualifying patient at any time, unless extra patients are parents, guardians or siblings. Caregiver registration mandatory. Past drug convictions will disqualify a caregiver for registration.

Connecticut Access Rating: Hard

Medical Dispensaries

Caregivers and patients can only obtain medical cannabis from licensed dispensaries. Connecticut has six dispensary facilities whose locations are available online[14] as of June 2015, and four producers. More on the way soon.

Patients must assign themselves to a dispensary facility and apply to re-assign to another dispensary. Cannabis is pharmaceutical-grade, lab-tested, labeled, pure and consistent.

11 http://www.cga.ct.gov/current/pub/chap_420f.htm.

12 https://www.biznet.ct.gov/AccountMaint/Login.aspx.

13 http://www.ct.gov/dcp.

14 http://www.ct.gov/dcp/cwp/view.asp?a=4287&q=548068.

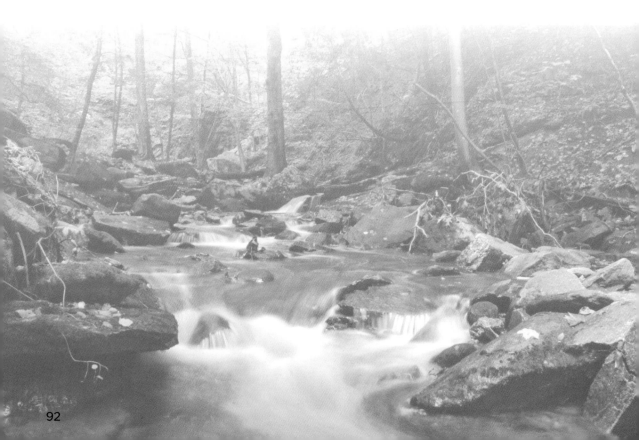

Washington, D.C. Access Rating: Medium

Recreational Legalization

Ballot Measure 71 legalized cannabis for all adults 21 and over, allowing them to possess up to two ounces, grow no more than six plants (with three or fewer being mature), transfer up to one ounce to another person 21 years or older, and use or sell accessories like pipes and growing mediums. It also legalized commercial farms and stores, but Congress is blocking their rollout.

Medical Law

Qualifying patients can obtain and use marijuana with a signed recommendation from a primary physician, and Washington, D.C., has licensed growers and stores. The District first enacted medical marijuana legislation[15] in 2010, but it was blocked by Congress until 2014. Rules[16] for the District's medical program were enacted in 2015.

Qualifying Conditions

HIV, AIDS, glaucoma, muscle spasms, multiple sclerosis, cancer, chemotherapy, azidothymidine or protease inhibitors, radiotherapy, and any "serious," "chronic" or "debilitating" conditions.

Limits

Qualifying patients and caregivers can have up to two ounces of dried flower bud.

Doctor's Recommendation

A licensed doctor or osteopath in the District may recommend medical cannabis if the doctor is in a bona fide physician-patient relationship, has completed a full assessment of the patient's medical history and current medical condition, including an in-person physical exam, has "responsibility for the ongoing care and treatment of the patient … not … limited to or for the primary purpose of the provision of medical marijuana," and has reviewed other approved medications that might provide relief, and is not the owner, director, officer, member, incorporator, agent or employee of a Dispensary or Cultivation Center. Physicians can fill out a request to access an electronic recommendation form[17].

ID Card

Mandatory. Database is confidential. You must be a D.C. resident, with proof of residence, qualifying illness or

Washington, D.C

Access Rating: Hard

treatment, formal doctor's recommendation filed with completed application[18] (online or in print) from the Department of Health. You'll need to include a recent passport-type photo, and a clear copy of a U.S., state or District photo ID as proof of identity, plus Physician Recommendation Number dated within 90 days of the application, and Social Security Number. Registration fee is $100, with a $25 renewal fee. There are 3,764 patients registered as of June 2015.[19]

Caregivers

Must be designated by patient, register with Department of Health, must not be caregiving for another, be at least 18 years of age, and never been convicted of possession or sale of a controlled substance. Caregivers must get a mandatory ID card by filling out a Caregiver Application Form[20] including two recent passport-type photos, and a clear copy of a U.S., state or District photo ID as proof of identity. Application fee is $100, with a $25 renewal. (There are reduced fees for caregivers making less than 200 percent of the federal poverty level). Background check and Social Security Number required.

Medical Dispensaries

There are five cultivation centers and three dispensaries that are listed on the Washington D.C.'s Department of Health website. Patients cannot visit multiple dispensaries.

---

15 http://doh.dc.gov/sites/default/files/dc/sites/doh/publication/attachments/Legal-Marijuana-Med-Treat-Amend-Act-2010_0.pdf.

16 http://doh.dc.gov/sites/default/files/dc/sites/doh/publication/attachments/Failure%20to%20open%20Emergency%20and%20Proposed%20effective.pdf.

17 https://octo.quickbase.com/db/biwy2t5h7?a=dbpage&pageID=7.

18 http://doh.dc.gov/sites/default/files/dc/sites/doh/publication/attachments/140610%20MMP%20Patient%20Application%20Instructions_0.pdf.

19 http://doh.dc.gov/sites/default/files/dc/sites/doh/publication/attachments/MMPProgramUpdateMemo1150629.pdf.

20 http://doh.dc.gov/sites/default/files/dc/sites/doh/publication/attachments/130611Caregiver%20applicationFINAL_1_0.pdf.

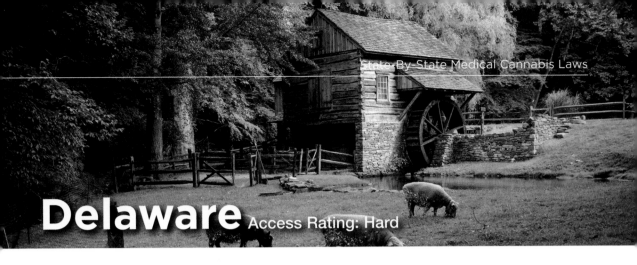

Delaware Access Rating: Hard

Medical Law [21]
Medical marijuana has been legal since 2011, with a tight, mandatory registration system for patients, caregivers, producers, and stores. Qualifying patients and caregivers also have discrimination protections with regard to jobs, education, housing, parenting, and medical care.

Qualifying Conditions
Cancer; HIV and AIDs; decompensated cirrhosis (hepatitis C); amyotrophic lateral sclerosis (Lou Gehrig's disease); agitation of Alzheimer's disease or the treatment of these conditions; severe post-traumatic stress disorder (PTSD); a chronic or debilitating disease causing cachexia or wasting syndrome; severe, chronic, intractable debilitating pain; intractable nausea; seizures; severe and persistent muscle spasms, including but not limited to those characteristic of multiple sclerosis.

Limits
Six ounces of usable cannabis per patient. No cultivation allowed.

Doctor's Recommendation
A primary care physician or a cannabinoid-specialized doctor can lawfully recommend marijuana.

ID Card
Mandatory. Apply by downloading and mailing in the application form [22]. Doctor fills out the physician certification component of the application. Annual fee $125. (Sliding scale for patients who demonstrate need.)

Caregivers
Must be 21 and older, not convicted of an excluded felony offense, and have no more than five patients. Patients designate caregivers on patient's application form, and caregiver submits a separate caregiver application [23].

Medical Dispensaries
Compassion centers are the only legal source of cannabis. The state's first Compassion Center at 37 Germay Drive in Wilmington opened June 26, 2015.

---

21 http://delcode.delaware.gov/title16/c049a/index.shtml.

22 http://dhss.delaware.gov/dph/hsp/files/mmppatientapplication.pdf.

23 http://dhss.delaware.gov/dph/hsp/files/mmpcaregiverapplication.pdf.

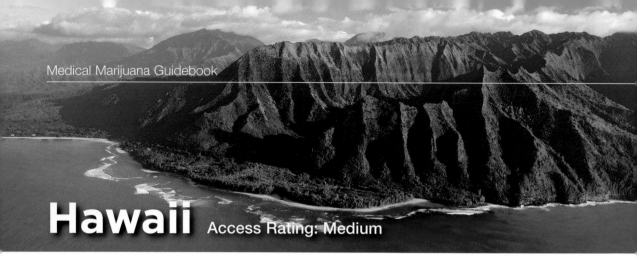

Hawaii Access Rating: Medium

Medical Law

Qualified, registered patients have the right to an affirmative defense in court during prosecution for certain marijuana crimes. Law enforcement can look up patient registration, providing extra protection from arrest. The Department of Health took over the unsatisfactory program from the police in 2015.[24]

Qualifying Conditions

Cachexia or wasting syndrome, severe pain, severe nausea, seizures, including epilepsy, severe and persistent muscle spasms, Crohn's disease, PTSD, or any other medical condition approved by the Department of Health.

Limits

Three ounces of usable cannabis and up to seven plants (three being mature).

Doctor's Recommendation

Doctors are the gateway to the Hawaii registry program, which is mandatory for legal protections. The Drug Policy Forum of Hawaii can assist you in finding a cannabis-specialized primary care physician.

You have to ask your primary care doctor to complete[25] an online application form that includes: completed Patient Applicant Certification[26],

(Minor Certification[27] if needed), Physician Certification[28] and if applicable, a Caregiver Certification[29] and a Grow Site Certification[30], along with a fee of $38.50.

The doctor submits the completed materials to the Medical Marijuana Registry online at https://medmj.ehawaii.gov/medmj/welcome.html. The program is obtuse. (email medicalmarijuana@doh.hawaii.gov to reach the program directly, or call 808-695-4620 for help).

Also, doctors must print out a hard copy of the entire completed Application Packet and mail it in to: Department of Health, Medical Marijuana Program, 4348 Waialae Avenue, #648, Honolulu, HI 96816

ID Card

Mandatory for patients and caregivers and obtained through primary care doctor. The Department of Health mails a patient's and caregiver's ID card to the doctor, who signs it and gives it to the patient. There were 12,005 registered patients in Hawaii as of 2013.

Caregivers

One patient per caregiver maximum, 18 years and older, who agrees to "undertake responsibility for managing the well-being of the qualifying patient with respect to the medical use of marijuana." Many caregivers will need to stop growing medicine by 2018, under a new dispensary bill HB 321.

Medical Dispensaries

A bill to allow 16 dispensaries passed in May 2015, and the first group of them may be open by July 2016. Contact the Drug Policy Forum of Hawaii for more info at http://dpfhi.org.

24 http://health.hawaii.gov/medicalmarijuana/.

25 http://health.hawaii.gov/medicalmarijuana/files/2014/11/CBD-002-Application-Instructions.pdf.

26 http://health.hawaii.gov/medicalmarijuana/files/2014/11/CBD-001ac-Patient-Certification-11.24.14.pdf.

27 http://health.hawaii.gov/medicalmarijuana/files/2014/11/CBD-001mc-Minor-Certification-11.24.14.pdf.

28 http://health.hawaii.gov/medicalmarijuana/files/2015/01/CBD-001pc-Physician-Certification-11.24.14.pdf.

29 http://health.hawaii.gov/medicalmarijuana/files/2014/11/CBD-001cc-Caregiver-Certification-11.24.14.pdf.

30 http://health.hawaii.gov/medicalmarijuana/files/2014/11/CBD-001gsc-Grow-Site-Certification-11.24.14.pdf.

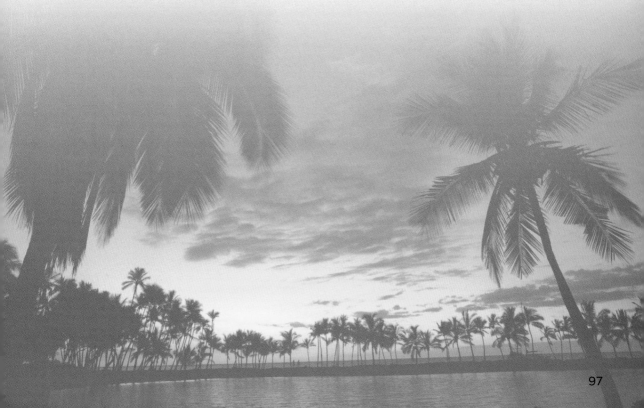

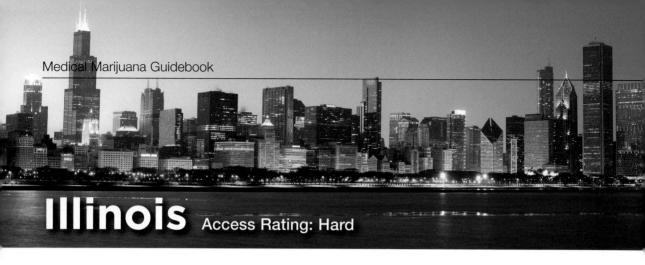

Illinois Access Rating: Hard

Medical Law

Illinois enacted a very strict medical cannabis law in 2013, HB 1, which immunizes patients from certain cannabis crimes, and calls for a statewide system of farms and stores.

Qualifying Conditions

Cancer, glaucoma, HIV/AIDS, hepatitis C, amyotrophic lateral sclerosis (ALS), Crohn's disease, Alzheimer's disease, cachexia/wasting syndrome, muscular dystrophy, fibromyalgia, spinal cord disease (including but not limited to arachnoiditis), Tarlov cysts, hydromyelia, syringomyelia, rheumatoid arthritis, fibrous dysplasia, traumatic brain injury and post-concussion syndrome, multiple sclerosis, Arnold-Chiari malformation, spinocerebellar ataxia (SCA), Parkinson's disease, Tourette's syndrome, myoclonus, dystonia, reflex sympathetic dystrophy (RSD), causalgia, CRPS (Complex Regional Pain Syndrome Type II), neurofibromatosis, chronic inflammatory demyelinating polyneuropathy, Sjogren's syndrome, lupus, interstitial cystitis, myasthenia gravis, hydrocephalus, nail patella syndrome or any other debilitating medical condition added by the Department of Public Health. Minors not allowed, except for those with epilepsy.

Limits

Up to 2.5 ounces of usable cannabis, unless waiver for more. No home cultivation allowed.

Doctor's Recommendation

You need a bona fide physician-patient relationship, a recent in-person exam, full assessment of medical history, including review of records for the last 12 months. Bona fide is defined as a relationship in which the physician has an "ongoing responsibility for the assessment, care and treatment of a patient's debilitating medical condition." Medical cannabis-specialized clinics are open in Illinois. The physician, not the patient, mails in a Physician Certification Form to: Illinois Department of Public Health, Division of Medical Cannabis, 535 West Jefferson St., Springfield, IL 62761-0001. About 2,600 patients have been approved by the state as of June 2015.

ID Card

Mandatory. Requires[31] written certification from their physician for the use of medical cannabis, Social Security Number, proof of residency, photo, clean record, $35 fee, fingerprint consent form, and signature. Patients and caregivers can submit medical cannabis registry applications online[32] or mail to:

Illinois Department of Public Health, Division of Medical Cannabis, 535 West Jefferson St. Springfield, IL 62761-0001. Requires a completed Patient Application Form[33], Caregiver Application Form[34] (if applicable), Physician Certification Form[35], Fingerprint Consent Form[36] (for federal background check), and $100 fee.

Caregivers

Must be 21 or over. One patient per caregiver. Cannot be convicted of an excluded offense (violent or felony drug crime, subject to waiver).

Medical Dispensaries

As of July 2015, Illinois is working to open up to 60 licensed dispensaries. Patients will self-assign to a particular district's or county's dispensaries.

---

31 http://www.dph.illinois.gov/sites/default/files/publications/publicationsmedical-cannabistop10medicalcannabis3.4.15.pdf.

32 https://medicalcannabispatients.illinois.gov/.

33 http://www.dph.illinois.gov/sites/default/files/forms/patient-application-form-080814.pdf.

34 http://www.dph.illinois.gov/sites/default/files/forms/caregiver-application-form-080814.pdf.

35 http://www.dph.illinois.gov/sites/default/files/forms/formsohpmmedical-cannabis-physician-written-certification.pdf.

36 https://docs.google.com/spreadsheets/d/1PJuqpsyAUi-74LJ1u0Q4sg1_gjlW1UcEQdfHND8Ohng/edit#gid=0.

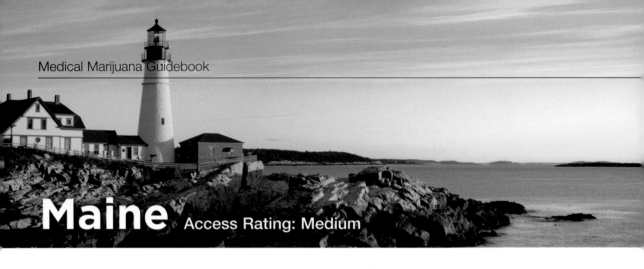

Maine Access Rating: Medium

Medical Law

Patients have protection from arrest for certain marijuana crimes if they have their original written certification from a doctor. Patients also enjoy protections from discrimination over school, employment, housing, and parental rights.

Qualifying Conditions

Cancer, glaucoma, positive status for human immunodeficiency virus, acquired immune deficiency syndrome, hepatitis C, amyotrophic lateral sclerosis, Crohn's disease, agitation of Alzheimer's disease, nail-patella syndrome or the treatment of these conditions, a chronic or debilitating disease or medical condition or its treatment that produces intractable pain (which is pain that has not responded to ordinary medical or surgical measures for more than 6 months), and a chronic or debilitating disease or medical condition or its treatment that produces one or more of the following: cachexia or wasting syndrome; severe nausea; seizures, including but not limited to those characteristic of epilepsy; or severe and persistent muscle spasms, including but not limited to those characteristic of multiple sclerosis.

Limits

Up to 2.5 ounces per qualified patient. Up to six mature plants per patient. You can't buy more than 2.5 ounces of marijuana from a dispensary in a 15-day period.

Doctor's Recommendation

Doctors can certify medical cannabis patients for the state registry online[37]. State registration of patients became mandatory in January 2015. Consulting physician approval required for doctor's approval of medical cannabis use for a minor.

ID Card

Mandatory. You obtain a Medical Cannabis Program card from the DHHS. Application is located online[38]. Requires copy of patient's current Maine driver's license or other Maine photo ID, patient's Physician Certification. No fee to register. Application materials can also be requested in written format by mailing a request to: Maine Medical Use of Marijuana Program, Division of Licensing and Regulatory Services, Department of Health and Human Services, 11 State House Station, Augusta, ME 04333.

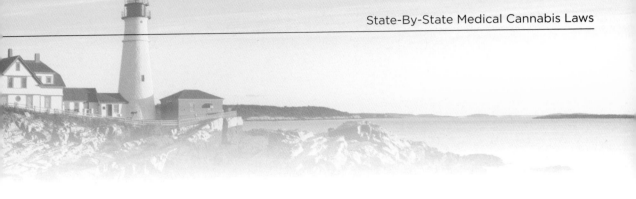

Caregivers

State registration[39] is mandatory. Can cultivate for patients. Secondary caregivers allowed. Five patients maximum per caregiver. Subject to background check and certain exclusions. $31 fee for background check. $300 cultivation fee per patient.

Medical Dispensaries

Maine has eight licensed dispensaries listed on the DHHS website[40]. You can find caregivers and dispensaries at online directories, including Medical Marijuana Caregivers of Maine[41].

---

37 https://www1.maine.gov/online/medmarijuana/index.html.

38 https://www1.maine.gov/dhhs/dlrs/mmm/application-material/Patient-Application.pdf.

39 http://www.maine.gov/dhhs/dlrs/mmm/documents/1-05-15-MMMP-Caregiver-Application2.pdf.

40 http://www.maine.gov/dhhs/dlrs/mmm/documents/Maine-Dispensaries-town-and-phone.pdf.

41 http://mmcm-online.org/index.php/for-patients/caregiver-directory.

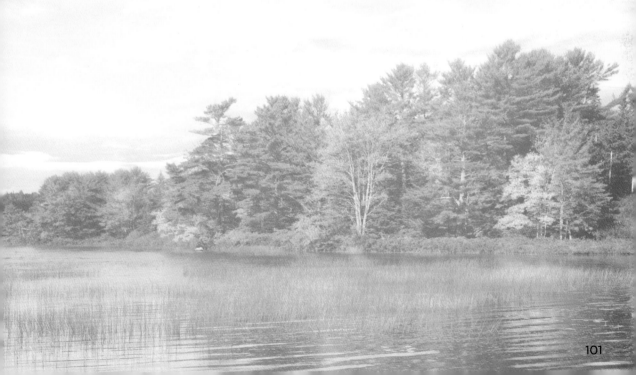

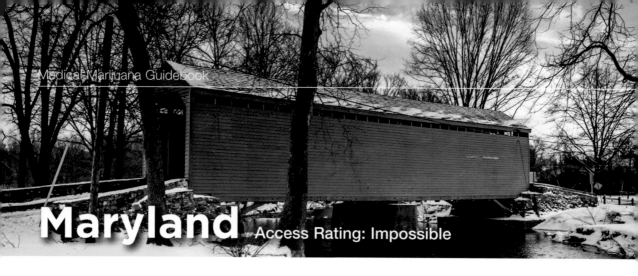

Maryland Access Rating: Impossible

Medical Law

Maryland has a form of limited medical cannabis decriminalization under five related bills. Patients have a limited affirmative defense in court against prosecution for certain cannabis crimes, and face a maximum $100 fine.[42] Their state system is only beginning to take shape.

Qualifying Conditions

"Debilitating medical condition" means a chronic or debilitating disease or medical condition or the treatment of a chronic or debilitating disease or medical condition that produces one or more of the following, as documented by a physician with whom the patient has a bona fide physician-patient relationship: cachexia or wasting syndrome; severe or chronic pain; severe nausea; seizures; severe and persistent muscle spasms; or any other condition that is severe and resistant to conventional medicine.

Limits

No specific possession limit, and determined by Commission. But generally no more than four ounces[43]. Maximum 36 grams of THC per month. No home-growing allowed.

Doctor's Recommendation

Only physicians who have active, unrestricted licenses in good standing with the Maryland Board of Physicians may be registered and may issue written certifications to patients with whom they have a "bona fide physician-patient relationship" where "the physician has ongoing responsibility for the assessment, care, and treatment of a patient's medical condition" and the physician has examined the patient, reviewed medical records, assessed the patient's medical history, maintains records on the patient, and will provide follow-up care to the patient as needed. Doctors will register the written certification on the Commission's website.

ID Card

Allows for adults as well as children with caregiver. Patients register online and then go to a doctor to obtain a "written certification." The actual physical ID Card is optional and $50.

Caregivers

Allowed under law, 21 or over. State residents only. Designated by patients. Subject to exclusions. One patient per caregiver.

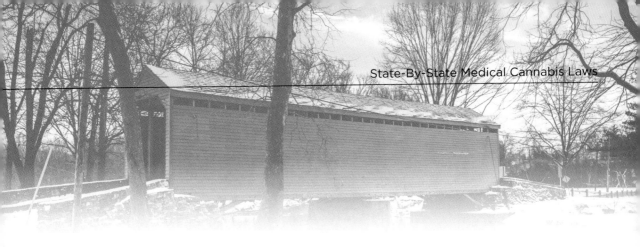

Medical Dispensaries

Dispensaries are not open in Maryland, but the state anticipates medical cannabis could be available to patients in the second half of 2016. Then patients can go to any dispensary. For more information, keep an eye on http://mmcc.maryland.gov/

42 http://mgaleg.maryland.gov/2013RS/chapters_noln/Ch_62_hb0180T.pdf.

43 http://mmcc.maryland.gov/pages/patients/patients_faq.aspx.

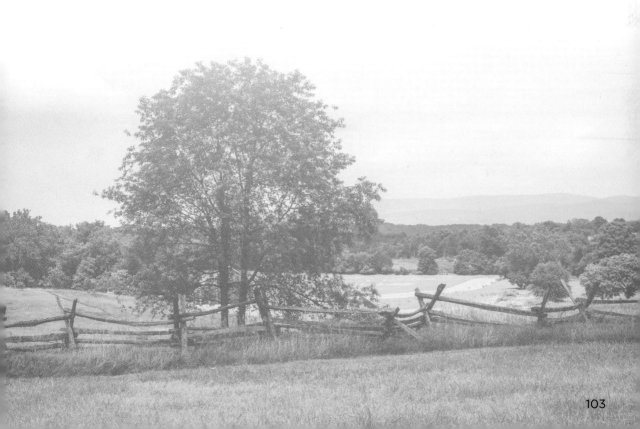

Massachusetts Access Rating: Hard

Medical Law

Massachusetts voted yes on Question 3 in 2012, and the state has been working toward a complete state-licensed medical cannabis system.

Qualifying Conditions

Cancer, glaucoma, HIV, AIDS, hepatitis C, amyotrophic lateral sclerosis (ALS), Crohn's disease, Parkinson's disease, multiple sclerosis, and other conditions as determined in writing by a qualifying patient's physician.

Limits

Up to 10 ounces of usable cannabis. No home cultivation (subject to hardship exception).

Doctor's Recommendation

You must make an appointment with your doctor to begin the registration process. If you are qualified, your provider will issue you a certification through the MMJ Online System[44]. Physicians must have a minimum of two Continuing Medical Education credits for the medical use of marijuana. Online directories like WeedMaps.com list many medical cannabis-specialized clinics.

ID Card

All patients must obtain an electronic certification from their physician and be registered with the Medical Use of Marijuana Program to possess marijuana for medical use. Your doctor issues you a certification and instructions on how to register through the MMJ Online System and a PIN. This PIN is required for you to register in the MMJ Online System. You will need Internet access, certain scanned documents, a valid form of ID, a photo of yourself, and a form of payment for the fee $50 (credit/debit/ETF).[45] Approved registrants receive a Medical Use of Marijuana Program ID Card. If you can't register online, a slower paper option is available. Massachusetts has 20,362 patients certified as of July 2015.

Caregivers

Ages 21 and over. Online registration mandatory.[46] You will need Internet access, scanned documents, a valid form of ID, a photo of yourself, and a form of payment for the fee $50 (credit/debit/ETF), and a PIN from your patient.

Medical Dispensaries

The first dispensaries are just starting to open in Massachusetts, with more scheduled to come online. For more info, see http://www.compassionforpatients.com.

44 http://www.mass.gov/eohhs/docs/dph/quality/medical-marijuana/mmj-system-registration-physician-step-by-step.pdf.\

45 http://www.mass.gov/eohhs/docs/dph/quality/medical-marijuana/mmj-system-registration-patient-step-by-step.pdf.

46 http://www.mass.gov/eohhs/docs/dph/quality/medical-marijuana/mmj-system-registration-caregiver-step-by-step.pdf.

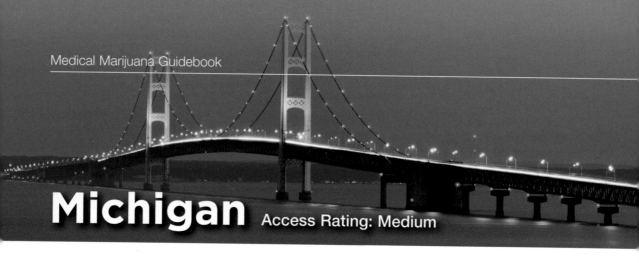

Michigan Access Rating: Medium

Medical Law

The Michigan Medical Marijuana Act of 2008 gives patients and their caregivers with a valid doctor's note an affirmative defense in court against prosecution for some cannabis crimes. Obtaining a state ID card further immunizes patients and caregivers from arrest for certain cannabis crimes. Dispensaries are illegal.

Qualifying Conditions

Alzheimer's disease, amyotrophic lateral sclerosis, cachexia or wasting syndrome, cancer, chronic pain, Crohn's disease, glaucoma, HIV or AIDS, hepatitis C, nail patella, nausea, post-traumatic stress disorder (PTSD), seizures, and severe and persistent muscle spasms.

Limits

Two and half ounces of usable cannabis. No more than 12 plants in an enclosed, locked facility or a greenhouse-type structure.

Doctor's Recommendation

You need a signed, complete Physician Certification Form from a Michigan state-licensed physician ("written certification") with whom you have a bonafide physician-patient relationship. The document states your debilitating medical condition(s) and that the physician has completed a full exam including your relevant medical history, and an in-person exam, and that it is the physician's professional opinion that the patient is likely to receive therapeutic or palliative benefit from the medical use of marijuana to treat or alleviate the patient's debilitating medical condition or symptoms associated with the debilitating medical condition.

ID Card

You get an ID card by downloading, printing out, completing and mailing in a patient application packet[47]. Make sure to have a copy of a valid ID, and a complete Physician Certification Form. Mail only one complete application and all required documentation in one envelope to: Michigan Medical Marijuana Program, P.O. Box 30083, Lansing, MI 48909. Make checks or money orders payable to: State of Michigan-MMMP ($60 patient fee, $25 caregiver). Minors have a separate but similar application where a caregiver as well as two doctor's signatures is necessary.[48] Michigan has about 100,000 registered patients.

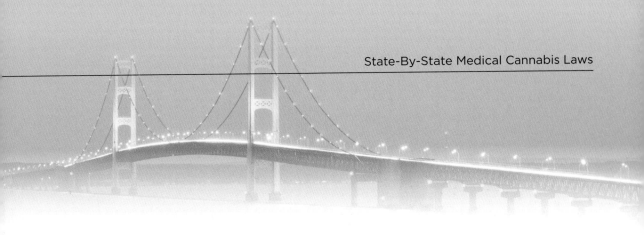

Caregivers

Yes, ages 21 and up, with no felony drug or violence convictions. One caregiver per patient. Up to five patients per caregiver.

Medical Dispensaries

No state-licensed dispensaries but regionally licensed ones and "compassion clubs." Lists of available dispensaries are online at directory sites like WeedMaps.com and Yelp.com.

---

47 http://www.michigan.gov/documents/lara/lara_BHCS_MMMP_Application_Packet_0115_478291_7.pdf.

48 http://www.michigan.gov/documents/lara/lara_BHCS_MMMP_MINOR_Application_Packet_0115_478522_7.pdf.

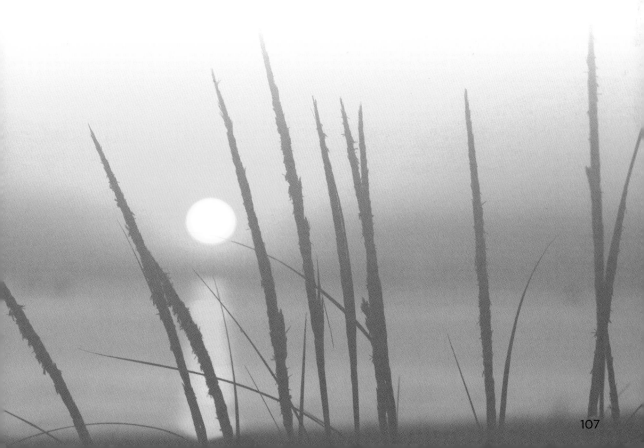

Minnesota Access Rating: Hard

Medical Law

Minnesota's medical marijuana law is one of the least helpful in the nation. It's very difficult to find a health practitioner willing to recommend the botanical. Patients cannot have caregivers, smoke raw flower buds, or cultivate their own plants. State-licensed cannabis outlets are open, however.

Qualifying Conditions

Cancer, glaucoma, HIV/AIDS, Tourette's syndorme, ALS, seizures/epilepsy, severe and persistent muscle spasms/MS, Crohn's disease, and terminal illness with a life expectancy of under one year.

Limits

Maximum 30-day supply per patient. Smoking not approved. Only formulations that are liquid, oil, and vaporizers of such extracts. No dried herb vaporization. No home cultivation.

Doctor's Recommendation

Three out of four Minnesota doctors are reportedly undecided or opposed to issuing medical cannabis certifications, so finding a specialist is more difficult. Doctors, physician assistants and advanced practice registered nurses must enroll in the Medical Cannabis Registry,[49] then log in to certify patients. Minnesota does not share any list of doctors participating in the program. Reports indicate 265 practitioners had signed up as of July 2015.

ID Card

Mandatory. You start by finding a doctor to certify you online, then you receive an email from the Office of Medical Cannabis with a link to register online. You're going to need basic contact information, government-issued ID, and a credit card to pay an annual registration fee of $200 ($50 for patients on Social Security disability, Supplemental Security Insurance, or enrolled in MinnesotaCare). You receive an email when your account is approved, then complete a self-reporting form in your online registry account. Next, you or your caregiver visits a Cannabis Patient Center where a pharmacist reviews your account, and recommends dosage and type. As of July 2015, 147 patients had been approved to obtain medical cannabis.[50]

Caregivers

Parents, legal guardians and caregivers can help with registration and medical cannabis pickup. Certified patients supply caregiver's email to registry. Caregiver signs up online via link, with contact info, government-issued ID,

and background check application form and fee ($15).

Medical Dispensaries
No retail facilities, but manufacturers should soon begin supplying patients.

Two are listed as open in Eagan and Minneapolis.[51] Eight total are scheduled to open by summer 2016.

49 https://apps.health.state.mn.us/cannabis/enrollment/health-care-practitioner/enroll-health-care-practitioner.xhtml.

50 http://www.health.state.mn.us/topics/cannabis/about/stats.html.

51 http://www.health.state.mn.us/topics/cannabis/patients/locations.html.

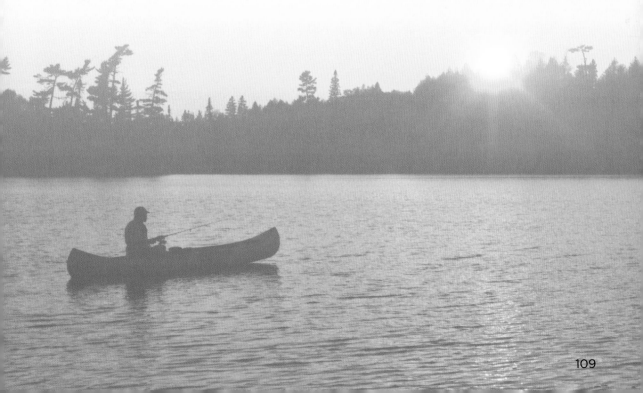

Montana Access Rating: Hard

Medical Law

Qualified patients and caregivers registered in the Montana system may not be arrested, prosecuted or penalized[52] for possession of certain amounts of marijuana and plants. Doctors also have protections to write cannabis recommendations.

Qualifying Conditions

Cancer; glaucoma; positive status for HIV/AIDS when the condition or disease results in symptoms that seriously and adversely affect the patient's health status; cachexia or wasting syndrome; severe, chronic pain that is persistent pain of severe intensity that significantly interferes with daily activities as documented by the patient's treating physician; intractable nausea or vomiting; epilepsy or intractable seizure disorder; multiple sclerosis; Crohn's disease; painful peripheral neuropathy; a central nervous system disorder resulting in chronic, painful spasticity or muscle spasms; admittance into hospice care.

Limits

Patients or their providers can have one ounce of usable marijuana, 12 seedlings, and four mature flowering plants.

Doctor's Recommendation

You have to get a state-licensed doctor or osteopath to complete a Physician Statement for a Debilitating Medical Condition[53]. Chronic pain diagnosis requires a separate form[54] and a second physician's signature.

ID Card

Mandatory. Requires state ID card. Non-refundable fee of $75 payable by check or money order. Download and complete an application packet[55], and be prepared to include a photocopy of a valid Montana driver's license or state ID, Physician Statement, signature of marijuana provider (if applicable), landlord permission form (if applicable). Mail to: DPHHS/MMP, P.O. BOX 202953, Helena, MT 59620 2953. Program is open to minors (with parent or guardian) using applicable forms.[56]

Caregivers

Patients can list a "provider" in their application and must include the signature of provider. Provider must complete and submit own packet[57].

Medical Dispensaries

None.

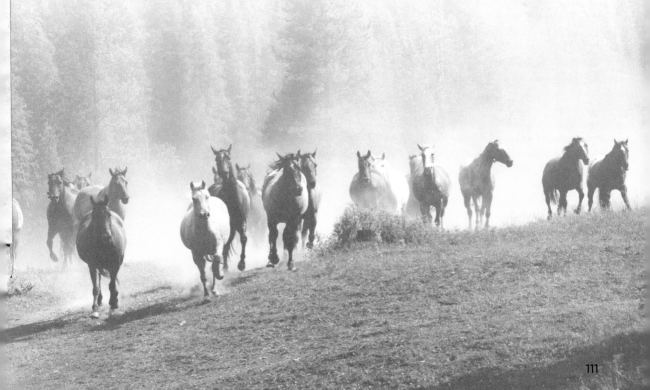

52 http://leg.mt.gov/bills/mca/50/46/50-46-319.htm.

53 http://dphhs.mt.gov/Portals/85/qad/documents/LicensureBureau/MarijuanaProgram/physiciansstatementcondition.pdf.

54 http://dphhs.mt.gov/Portals/85/qad/documents/LicensureBureau/MarijuanaProgram/chronicpainphysicianstmnt.pdf.

55 http://dphhs.mt.gov/Portals/85/qad/documents/LicensureBureau/MarijuanaProgram/patientapplication.pdf.

56 http://dphhs.mt.gov/Portals/85/qad/documents/LicensureBureau/MarijuanaProgram/patientapplicationminor.pdf.

57 http://dphhs.mt.gov/Portals/85/qad/documents/LicensureBureau/MarijuanaProgram/providermipapplication.pdf.

Nevada Access Rating: Medium

Medical Law

Nevada has enacted multiple laws that give patients, caregivers and their doctors a shield in court against prosecution for certain marijuana crimes, as well establish a mandatory state registry, and a system of state-licensed dispensaries.

Qualifying Conditions

Cancer; glaucoma; AIDS; severe, persistent nausea or cachexia resulting from these or other chronic or debilitating medical conditions; epilepsy and other disorders characterized by seizure; multiple sclerosis and other disorders characterized by muscular spasticity; or other conditions approved pursuant to law for such treatment.

Limits

Patients and their caregivers can possess no more than 2.5 ounces in a single 14-day period and grow no more than seven plants (three mature)[58].

Doctor's Recommendation

Any doctor of medicine (MD) or doctor of osteopathy (DO) licensed in Nevada can recommend a patient for the program. You can go online to find cannabis-specialized doctors in Nevada. You give them the Attending Physician's Statement form for them to fill out and give back to you.

ID Card

Mandatory. Send in a printed, complete written request form[59] for an application along with a check or money order via mail to: Nevada Division of Public and Behavioral Health, ATTN: Medical Marijuana Division, 4150 Technology Way, Suite 104, Carson City, NV 89706 ($25 request application fee). The state mails you the application forms and you fill them out and mail them back with a $75 ID card fee. Application requires written, signed Physician Statement recommending cannabis, and two notarized forms. State sends written notice of approval to patient (or requests fingerprints for deeper background check), and then patients go to approved DMV location to receive their Medical Marijuana Patient or Caregiver card. As of May 2015, there were 9,345 active patient cards.[60]

Caregivers

Yes. Include caregiver information in patient application request form, and patient application packet. One patient per caregiver. State sends written notice of approval to caregiver.

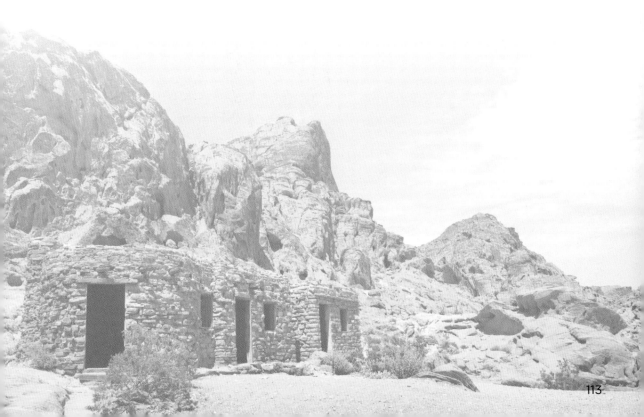

Medical Dispensaries

Yes. Nevada in 2015 opened its first state-licensed medical cannabis dispensaries. Nevada recognizes out-of-state patients' recommendations if they match any of Nevada's qualifying conditions.

---

58 http://www.health.nv.gov/MedicalMarijuana/ProgramFacts.pdf.

59 http://health.nv.gov/MedicalMarijuana/MMRRequest.pdf.

60 http://www.health.nv.gov/MedicalMarijuana/Reports/2015/MMP_May_2015.pdf.

New Hampshire

Medical Law

House Bill 573[61] in 2013 exempts certain individuals from prosecution for certain cannabis-related crimes.

Qualifying Conditions

ALS, Alzheimer's disease, cachexia, cancer, chemotherapy-induced anorexia, chronic pancreatitis, Crohn's disease, elevated intraocular pressure, epilepsy, glaucoma, hepatitis C (currently receiving antiviral treatment), HIV/AIDS, lupus, moderate to severe vomiting, multiple sclerosis, muscular dystrophy, nausea, Parkinson's disease, persistent muscle spasms, seizures, severe pain (that has not responded to previously prescribed medication), spinal cord injury or disease, traumatic brain injury, and wasting syndrome.

Limits

Two ounces usable cannabis[62]. No home-growing.

Doctor's Recommendation

Patients need to find a licensed physician to prescribe drugs, and who possesses certification from the United States Drug Enforcement Administration to prescribe controlled substances or an advanced practice registered nurse licensed and form a "provider-patient relationship" of at least three months in length that includes an in-person exam, history, diagnosis, and a treatment plan appropriate for the licensee's medical specialty. Then, obtain a "Written certification" of a qualifying medical condition for use in applying for a registry identification card. (The three-month requirement is subject to waiver for sudden onset of illness.) The date of issuance and the patient's qualifying medical condition, symptoms or side effects, the certifying provider's name, medical specialty, and signature shall be specified on the written certification.

ID Card

Mandatory. State has begun accepting patient applications. Application will require passport-sized photo, contact info, signed statement, designated caregiver (if applicable) and designated alternative treatment center[63]. Check for updates at the state's health department website.[64]

Caregivers

Yes. Age 21 or over. No more than five patients per caregiver (unless 50 miles from nearest dispensary, then it's nine patients). State began accepting patient applications in late 2015. Application will require passport-sized photo, contact info, signed statement, designated

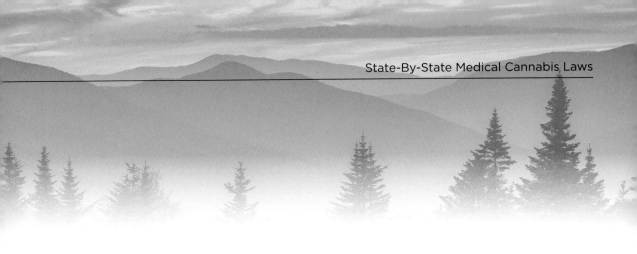

caregiver (if applicable) and designated alternative treatment center.[65] Background check including fingerprints will be required.

Medical Dispensaries

Yes, but no more than four dispensaries will be open in New Hampshire. As of April 2016, the state was working to open its first "Alternative Treatment Centers."

---

61 http://www.gencourt.state.nh.us/rsa/html/X/126-X/126-X-1.htm.

62 http://www.gencourt.state.nh.us/rsa/html/X/126-X/126-X-2.htm.

63 http://www.gencourt.state.nh.us/rsa/html/X/126-X/126-X-4.htm.

64 http://www.dhhs.state.nh.us/oos/tcp/.

65 http://www.gencourt.state.nh.us/rsa/html/X/126-X/126-X-4.htm.

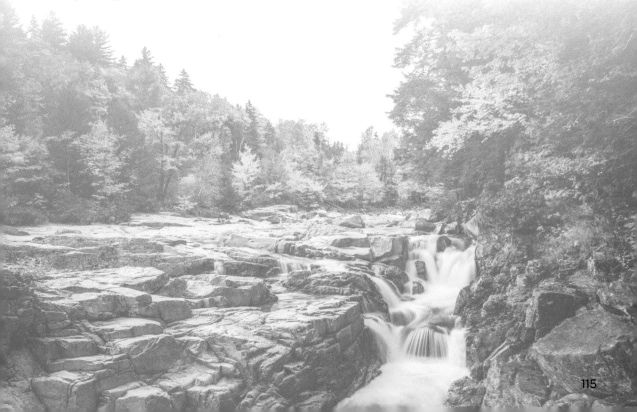

New Jersey Access Rating: Hard

Medical Law

New Jersey has enacted[66] a tightly controlled state-level medical cannabis system[67] with a few stores, a select group of registered doctors and a couple licensed cannabis farms. Registered patients and caregivers are protected[68] from arrest, prosecution, property forfeiture, and other penalties associated with certain marijuana crimes.

Qualifying Conditions

Seizure disorder including epilepsy, intractable skeletal muscular spasticity, glaucoma; severe or chronic pain, severe nausea or vomiting, cachexia, or wasting syndrome resulting from HIV/AIDS or cancer; amyotrophic lateral sclerosis (Lou Gehrig's disease), multiple sclerosis, terminal cancer, muscular dystrophy, or inflammatory bowel disease, including Crohn's disease; terminal illness, if the physician has determined a prognosis of less than 12 months of life or any other medical condition or its treatment that is approved by the Department of Health and Senior Services.

Limits

Two ounces per month. No home cultivation.

Doctor's Recommendation

Only doctors registered[70] with the state's program can make recommendations. Ask your doctor if they are registered, or seek out a cannabis-specialized clinician in New Jersey by searching the state's online directory. There are 325 active physicians in the program and you can look them up online on the state's health website[71]. Your doctor submits an "Attending Physician Statement" to the state, gets a Patient Reference Number, and gives you both the statement and the number for use in your online application. Recommendations last up to 90 days.

ID Card

Mandatory. Online registration[72]. Supply all required info and Reference Number and Physician Statement. Prepare to upload scanned photographs and documents, including passport-style photo, state ID, proof of residency, caregiver photo, ID, and proof of residency (if applicable). The program contacts you to complete the application and pay a $200 fee ($20 fee with proof of government assistance). Minors allowed with caregiver.

Caregivers

Yes. $200 fee, plus background check fee (includes fingerprints). One patient only. Patient adds caregiver, with similar documents required. Caregiver also applies separately.[73]

Medical Dispensaries

Allowed, but no more than six. Five are operational[74]. Patients must obtain all medicine from treatment center.

---

66 http://www.state.nj.us/health/medicalmarijuana/documents/cumma_ammendments_9_13.pdf.

67 http://www.state.nj.us/health/medicalmarijuana/documents/final_rules.pdf.

68 http://www.njleg.state.nj.us/2008/Bills/PL09/307_.HTM.

69 http://www.state.nj.us/health/medicalmarijuana/documents/annual_report_2014.pdf.

70 http://www.state.nj.us/health/medicalmarijuana/eligibility.shtml.

71 http://www.state.nj.us/health/medicalmarijuana/find_phy_pat.shtml.

72 https://njmmp.nj.gov/njmmp/jsp/patientRegProcess.jsp.

73 http://www.state.nj.us/health/medicalmarijuana/what_caregiver.shtml.

74 http://www.state.nj.us/health/medicalmarijuana/find_atc_pat.shtml.

New Mexico Access Rating: Hard

Medical Law

New Mexico has had a medical marijuana law since 2007, The Lynn and Erin Compassionate Use Act, but its implementation has been heavy handed. Registered patients and caregivers can't be arrested for certain cannabis crimes[75], but lengthy background checks are required to grow, and "nonprofit producers" (not dispensaries) are in short supply. New Mexico patients say the program underserves the state. As of June 2015, there were 15,625 active patients[76] and 23 nonprofit producers in a state of 2.1 million residents.

Qualifying Conditions

Cancer; glaucoma; multiple sclerosis; damage to the nervous tissue of the spinal cord, with objective neurological indication of intractable spasticity; epilepsy; HIV/AIDS; admission into hospice care; severe chronic pain (with objective proof, written certification of unremitting severe chronic pain condition, written by pain specialist in expertise in the disease causing the pain); peripheral neuropathy; intractable nausea/vomiting; severe anorexia/cachexia; hepatitis C infection; Crohn's disease; post-traumatic stress disorder (PTSD); inflammatory autoimmune-mediated arthritis; amyotrophic lateral sclerosis (Lou Gehrig's disease); inclusion body myositis; spasmodic torticollis (cervical dystonia); Parkinson's disease; Huntington's disease; ulcerative colitis; and such other conditions as the secretary may approve.[77] Minors allowed with parent or guardian as caregiver.

Limits

Six ounces every three months per patient or caregiver. For licensed personal growers, four mature female plants and 12 seedlings.[78]

Doctor's Recommendation

Your cannabis-specialized doctor fills out and signs a Medical Certification Form[79], which you add to your ID card application. Medical doctors (MD), doctors of osteopathy (DO), nurse practitioners (NP), and most mid-level medical providers can write certifications.

ID Card

Mandatory. Involves downloading and printing application[80] including a Medical Certification Form — including copies of medical records are a bonus — and a Medical Information Release, plus notes from the doctor, a valid New Mexico photo ID, and a separate form[81] for a Personal Production License, if you want to grow it. Mail it all to: Department of Health, Medical Cannabis Program, 1190 St. Francis Dr., Suite S3400, Santa Fe, NM 87505. No enrollment fee. Approved applicants are sent a confidential list of producers.

Caregivers

Yes, with mandatory registration[82]. Requires patient and doctor signatures, and federal background check.

Medical Dispensaries

Non-profit producers may operate with license, grow no more than 150 plants and sell extracts no stronger than 70 percent THC. There are currently 23 licensed producers.[83] The New Mexico Department of Health plans on adding 12 more producers.

75 http://164.64.110.239/nmac/parts/title07/07.034.0003.htm.

76 http://nmhealth.org/publication/view/report/1549/.

77 http://nmhealth.org/publication/view/help/132/.

78 http://164.64.110.239/nmac/parts/title07/07.034.0004.htm.

79 http://nmhealth.org/publication/view/form/135/.

80 http://nmhealth.org/publication/view/form/135/.

81 http://nmhealth.org/publication/view/form/136/.

82 http://nmhealth.org/publication/view/form/133/.

83 http://nmhealth.org/news/information/2014/2/?view=41.

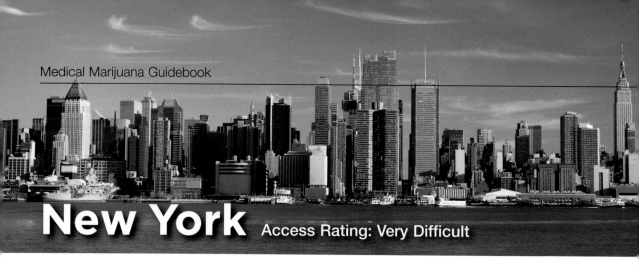

New York Access Rating: Very Difficult

Medical Law

New York's nascent, tightly controlled statewide system of medical cannabis licensing is nascent, and improvements will be slow in coming. No smoking is allowed in the Compassionate Care Act. Certified patients and caregivers, doctors and the industry are not subject to arrest. The certification process launched December 2015.[84] Disabilities protection laws apply to patients.[85]

Qualifying Conditions

Cancer, HIV, AIDS, ALS, multiple sclerosis, spinal cord damage resulting in spasticity, epilepsy, inflammatory bowel disease, neuropathies, Huntington's disease, cachexia/wasting, severe or chronic pain, severe nausea, severe or persistent muscle spasms.

Limits

Set by the Commissioner, and to not exceed a 30-day supply of the dosage.

Doctor's Recommendation

Doctors must first take an online course[86] and register with the program. Only then can a practitioner write a "patient certification" with an authorized medical brand and form, administration method, dosage, and amount of doses (less than a 30-day supply). A state Commissioner must approve any form of medical marijuana doctors recommend.

ID Card

Mandatory, and online.[87] $50 fee.

Caregivers

Yes with accepted application. Applications became available in December 2015. Patients may designate up to two caregivers during registration. After the patient's application is approved, designated caregiver(s) must register with the Department.

Medical Dispensaries

Twenty "registered organizations"[88] are called for to grow and sell cannabis. As of April 2016, 43 businesses had submitted applications to become eligible to grow and distribute medical cannabis. The first five were announced in July. The system will be ready when the Commissioner of Health and the Superintendent of State Police certifies it.

---

84 http://www.health.ny.gov/regulations/medical_marijuana/patients
85 http://assembly.state.ny.us/leg/?bn=A06357E&term=2013&Summary=Y&Actions=Y&Votes=Y&Memo=Y&Text=Y.
86 http://www.health.ny.gov/publications/1065.pdf
87 http://www.health.ny.gov/regulations/medical_marijuana/patients
88 http://www.health.ny.gov/regulations/medical_marijuana/application/selected_applicants.htm

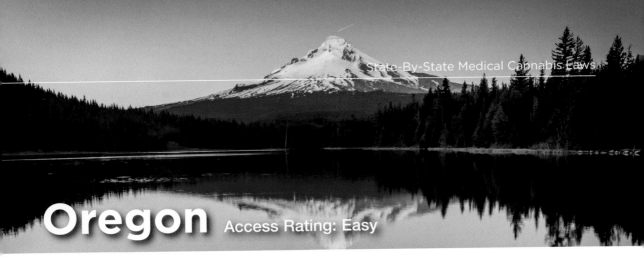

Oregon Access Rating: Easy

Recreational Legalization

Yes. Oregon legalized cannabis for all adults ages 21 and over in 2014 with Measure 91. Those adults can carry up to eight dried ounces of cannabis, and grow up to four plants. The state is in the process of licensing commercial growers and store operators in 2016.

Medical Law

Available since 1998, it's one of the most accessible and well developed in the country. Oregon's medical program runs in parallel with its recreational one. There were 73,605 patients, 35,864 caregivers[89] and 46,292 growers in the state program as of July 2015.[90]

Qualifying Conditions

Cancer, glaucoma, Alzheimer's disease agitation, HIV/AIDS, PTSD, cachexia, severe pain, severe nausea, seizures, epilepsy, muscle spasms, multiple sclerosis.

Limits

A qualified patient can have up to 24 ounces, and six mature plants and 18 seedlings.

Doctor's Recommendation

Doctors who will write a physician's statement are plentiful in Oregon, and there are 1,694 physicians associated with the program. Doctors fill out the state Attending Physician's Statement form[91], or a simple regular recommendation with your qualifying condition; a statement that medical marijuana may relieve the symptoms or effect of your qualifying condition; doctor's signature; and date. You include the statement or recommendation with application for the state program.

ID Card

Mandatory. OMMP Application Form[92] requires: Physician's Statement, copies of valid ID-like Driver's License, state ID card, passport, $200 fee (discounts available), and $50 grow site fee (if applicable). Minors allowed with caregiver. Send in complete forms with attachments by certified mail to: OHA/OMMP, P.O. Box 14450, Portland, OR 97293-0450; or drop it in the box on the first floor of the Portland State Office Building at 800 N.E. Oregon St., Portland, Oregon 97232-2162. Annual renewal required.

Caregivers

Yes, with completed caregiver section of patient application. Can have more than one patient. Most have no more than two, but one had 53 patients in 2015.

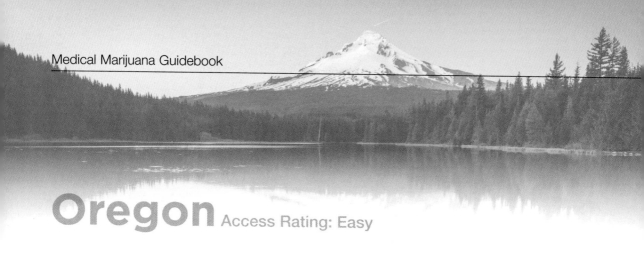

Oregon Access Rating: Easy

Medical Dispensaries

Registered patients must obtain cannabis from licensed dispensaries, grow it themselves, or have a caregiver grow it. Oregon has 417 registered dispensaries and they are listed in a state directory[93] on the state's website. Retail stores are set to open in 2016.

---

89 http://public.health.oregon.gov/DiseasesConditions/ChronicDisease/MedicalMarijuanaProgram/Documents/ed-materials/ommp_stats_snapshot.pdf.

90 http://public.health.oregon.gov/DiseasesConditions/ChronicDisease/MedicalMarijuanaProgram/Documents/ed-materials/ResidencySummary.pdf.

91 http://public.health.oregon.gov/DiseasesConditions/ChronicDisease/MedicalMarijuanaProgram/Documents/ommp-attending-physicians-statement.pdf.

92 http://public.health.oregon.gov/DiseasesConditions/ChronicDisease/MedicalMarijuanaProgram/Documents/application.pdf.

93 http://www.oregon.gov/oha/mmj/Pages/directory.aspx.

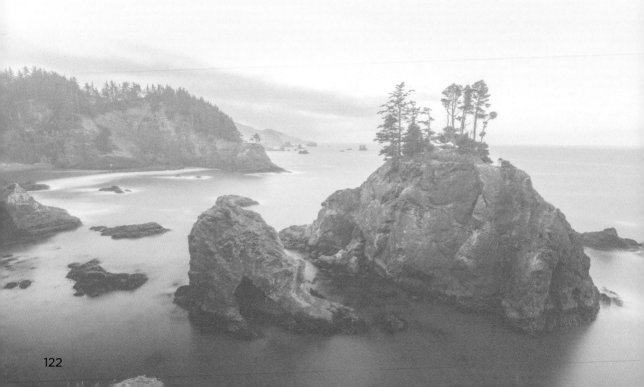

Rhode Island Access Rating: Hard

Medical Law

Rhode Island has a small, understaffed, heavily regulated, state-licensed medical cannabis system. Registered state medical marijuana program cardholders are not subject to arrest under the The Edward O. Hawkins and Thomas C. Slater Medical Marijuana Act[94]. There were 4,849 active patients and 3,415 caregivers in the program as the last reporting period (January 2013)[95]. Registered patients have certain housing, employment and education protections against discrimination.

Qualifying Conditions

Cancer, glaucoma, HIV/AIDS, hepatitis C, cachexia/wasting, severe debilitating chronic pain, severe nausea, seizures, epilepsy, muscle spasms, multiple sclerosis, Crohn's disease, Alzheimer's disease agitation.

Limits

Up to 2.5 ounces and 12 plants per patient. Cardholders can collectively cultivate.

Doctor's Recommendation

Have your doctor fill out a Practitioner Form[96] and include it with your application form. You must have a bonafide doctor patient relationship, including a recent in-person exam, review of medical records, etc.

ID Card

Mandatory. Download and complete Application Form[97] and include completed, signed Practitioner Form, $100 check to "RI General Treasurer," proof of residency like copy of a driver's license, state ID, or gas or electric bill. Minors allowed with caregiver. Mail packet to: Rhode Island, Office of Health Professionals Regulation, Medical Marijuana Program, Room 104 - 3 Capitol Hill, Providence, RI 02908-5097.

Caregivers

Yes. Ages 21 and over. Can have up to five patients. Maximum 24 plants. Patient can designate up to two on patient application form. Must obtain a National Criminal Records Check (NCRC). Disqualifications include some felony convictions. Fingerprints will be taken.

Medical Dispensaries

Patients can self-assign during application to up to two state-licensed Compassion Centers. There are currently three in the state.

---

94 http://webserver.rilin.state.ri.us/Statutes/TITLE21/21-28.6/INDEX.HTM.

95 http://www.health.ri.gov/publications/programreports/MedicalMarijuana2013.pdf.

96 http://www.health.ri.gov/forms/registration/MedicalMarijuanaPractitionerForm.pdf.

97 http://www.health.ri.gov/forms/registration/MedicalMarijuanaNewApplication.pdf.

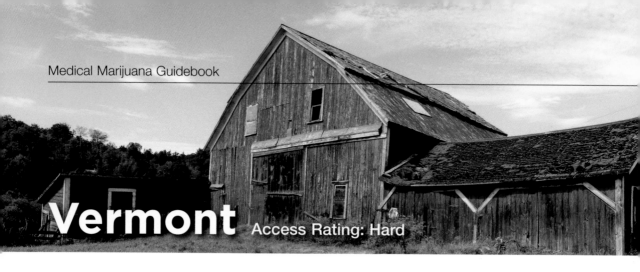

Vermont Access Rating: Hard

Medical Law

Since being enacted in 2007, Vermont has a narrow in scope, limited in access medical cannabis system with 1,754 patients[98][99] in 2015 and state-licensed dispensaries capped at a total of four[100] — for a population of well over 600,000. But registered patients, caregivers, growers and sellers are immune from arrest for certain cannabis crimes.

Qualifying Conditions

Cancer, multiple sclerosis, HIV, AIDS, chronic intractable cachexia or wasting, pain, nausea, or seizures.[101]

Limits

Registered patients or their caregivers can have two mature plants, seven immature ones, and two ounces of usable cannabis.

Doctor's Recommendation

Patients report being frustrated[102] trying to find a physician, physician's assistant, naturopath or Registered Nurse (APRN) to complete a Health Care Professional Verification Form[103]. You have to have a six-month doctor-patient relationship or a terminal illness; or cancer with distant metastases; or AIDS. There is an allowance for "recent or sudden onset" of a disease or symptom.

ID Card

Download and complete a Registered Patient Application[104], and include the completed and signed Health Care Professional Verification Form, electronic file of passport-style photograph to DPS.VTMR@state.vt.us, and a $50 non-refundable fee. Minors can apply with parent or guardian. Mail it to: Department of Public Safety, Marijuana Registry, 103 South Main St., Waterbury, VT 05671-2101. Notary required.

Caregivers

Yes. Only care for one patient per caregiver. Fill out caregiver portion[105] of patient's application and include a $50 check to the Department of Public Safety. Also, send a passport-style photo via email to DPS.VTMR@state.vt.us. Patients can register two caregivers.[106] A criminal background check of your name includes FBI records.

Medical Dispensaries

Patients can designate a dispensary, but forget about growing it by themselves or by a caregiver. There are four

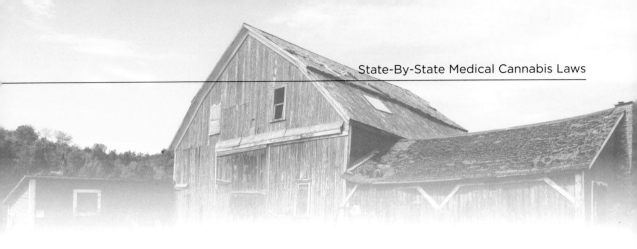

(capped) registered dispensaries open in Vermont: Champlain Valley Dispensary in Burlington; Vermont Patients Alliance in Montpelier; Rutland County Organics in Brandon; and Southern Vermont Wellness in Brattleboro. They're open by appointment only.

98 http://vcic.vermont.gov/sites/vcic/files/Patient%20and%20caregiver%20diagram%2020150325.pdf.

99 http://vcic.vermont.gov/sites/vcic/files/County_Map_March_25_2015.pdf.

100 http://vcic.vermont.gov/sites/vcic/files/Vermont%20Rules%202012.pdf.

101 http://vcic.vermont.gov/sites/vcic/files/Vermont%20Rules%202012.pdf.

102 http://vcic.vermont.gov/sites/vcic/files/Marijuana%20Oversight%20Committee%20Annual%20Report%2020150112.pdf.

103 http://vcic.vermont.gov/sites/vcic/files/Health%20Care%20Professional%20Form%202015-01.pdf.

104 http://vcic.vermont.gov/sites/vcic/files/Patient%20Application%202015-05.pdf.

105 http://vcic.vermont.gov/sites/vcic/files/Caregiver%20Application%202015.pdf.

106 http://vcic.vermont.gov/sites/vcic/files/Patient%20Application%202015-05.pdf.

Washington Access Rating: Easy

Recreational Legalization

Adults 21 and over are allowed up to an ounce of usable marijuana and access to state-licensed dispensaries — all part of Initiative 502[107], which voters passed in 2012. Dozens of stores are open, and more are coming. The state has authorized 2.9 million square-feet of cannabis fields. No home-growing allowed, which is part of why the medical system remains attractive to some residents.

Medical Law

Washington has had a relatively open medical cannabis system, starting in 1998[108], just two years after California. Washington's medical system is coming under tighter rules[109] amid the parallel recreational system. Personal limits are going down. Caregiving limits are shrinking. Unlicensed dispensaries are being deemed illegal. Registered patients pay no sales tax, but will have to jump through more hoops than recreational buyers.

Qualifying Conditions

Cancer, HIV, PTSD, epilepsy, spasticity, intractable pain, nausea, vomiting, wasting appetite loss, cramping, seizures, muscle spasms[110], glaucoma, Crohn's disease, hepatitis C, anorexia.

Limits

Up to 24 ounces of usable marijuana. No more than 15 plants. Those limits are decreasing on July 1, 2016, to six ounces and four plants for patients with a doctor's note but no registration.[111] Registered patients are allowed up to eight ounces, six plants, and access to retail stores.

Doctor's Recommendation

You get a doctor to fill out a written, signed recommendation and that's it. You're done. However, beginning in July 2016, all new authorizations must be written on a form developed by the department and printed on tamper-resistant paper. Here is the most recent form.[112] Cannabis-specialized clinicians are widely available in Washington and can be found in online directories like Yelp.com. Under new rules, doctors who write more than 30 authorizations per month must report doing so, could face increased scrutiny, and cannot solely issue medical marijuana authorizations.

ID Card

Not mandatory to raise an affirmative defense in court.[113] Form to apply for card is available at www.doh.wa.gov. Beginning July 1, 2016, registered patients enjoy greater limits, access, and rights than non-registered patients.

Caregivers
Yes. Washington has had a very loose caregiver program that only requires caregivers be designated in writing. Ages 21 and over. Growing cooperatives of up to four people allowed under new rules.

Medical Dispensaries
Washington has had a thriving medical dispensary industry that's facing new pressure amid a parallel recreational industry. Dispensaries were never technically legal, and soon patients will be able to buy at the licensed recreational stores, without recreational taxes. You can find dispensaries aplenty in online directories like WeedMaps.com. By July 1, 2016, all producers, processors and stores must be licensed by the Liquor Control Board, and supplies will be tested for potency and safety.

107 http://sos.wa.gov/_assets/elections/initiatives/i502.pdf.

108 https://www.sos.wa.gov/elections/initiatives/text/i692.pdf.

109 http://lawfilesext.leg.wa.gov/biennium/2015-16/Pdf./Bills/Session%20Laws/Senate/5052-S2.SL.pdf.

110 http://app.leg.wa.gov/rcw/default.aspx?cite=69.51A.010.

111 http://www.doh.wa.gov/YouandYourFamily/Marijuana/MedicalMarijuana/GeneralFrequentlyAskedQuestions.

112 http://www.doh.wa.gov/Portals/1/Documents/Pubs/630123.pdf.

113 http://app.leg.wa.gov/rcw/default.aspx?cite=69.51A&full=true#69.51A.043.

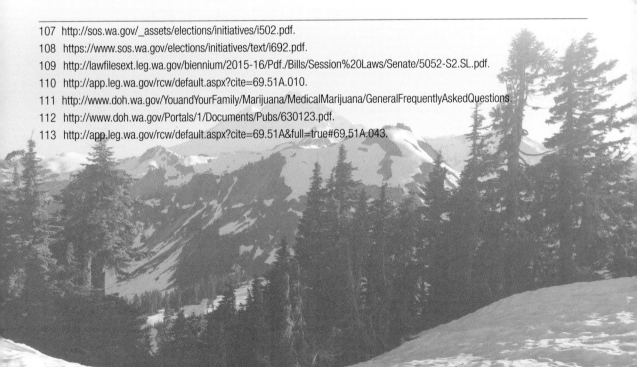

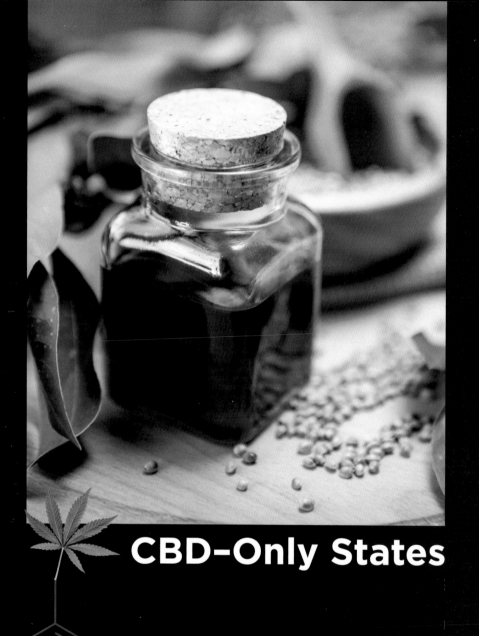

CBD–Only States

Alabama Access Rating: Virtually Impossible

Medical Law

Alabama has a CBD-only medical marijuana law passed in 2014 that allows a handful of catastrophic epilepsy patients access to a CBD-only oil made by GW Pharmaceuticals.

Qualifying Conditions

Catastrophic epilepsy.

Limits

Only state-approved clinical trial patients can possess CBD, and there are about 10 such patients as of July 2015. GW Pharmaceuticals supplies the CBD-only oil, which is taken orally.

Doctor's Recommendation

Only a few doctors at the University of Alabama-Birmingham Department of Neurology could potentially recommend CBD-only medication. Prospective patients must submit cover letter, checklist, referral letter from primary treating neurologist, and medical record information. Templates of the checklist and referral letter are online.[114] Extensive medical records required, including: history; brain MRI and electrocardiogram (ECG); video/EEG; documentation of failed epilepsy drugs; documentation of brain implantation; report of corpus callostomy or other surgery; documentation of seizure calendar for at least three months; and proof of Alabama residency. All documentation should be mailed via the U.S. Postal Service (email will not be accepted/considered) to the following address: Attn: CBD Program Manager, 1720 7th Avenue South. Sparks Center, 339C, Birmingham, AL 35233.

ID Card

No state system. You contact the university to request an application packet.[115]

Caregivers

No.

Medical Dispensaries

No

---

114 http://www.uab.edu/medicine/neurology/research/uab-cannabidiol-program.

115 http://www.uab.edu/medicine/neurology/research/uab-cannabidiol-program.

Florida
Access Rating: Impossible

Medical Law

Florida has a limited medical cannabis law[116] and a system that's not serving patients. The Compassionate Medical Cannabis Act of 2014 requires cannabis flowers have only trace amounts of THC, and more than 10 percent CBD. Only state-licensed stores and growers can provide it, but those growers and stores are limited. UnitedForCare and other organizations are working toward fully legalizing medical cannabis, as well as ending prohibition for adults 21 and over.

Qualifying Conditions

Cancer, chronic seizures, severe and persistent muscle spasms.

Limits

Dried flowers that are less than 0.8 percent THC and greater than 10 percent CBD, of whatever amount "ordered" by a physician. No smoking allowed. No home-growing.

Doctor's Recommendation

Requires exam, history review and diagnosis from medical, allopathic, and osteopathic doctors who then order medical cannabis for patients. Doctors have to take eight hours of coursework on recommending low-THC cannabis before they can order it for a patient on the state registry. The state's Health Department website maintains a list of physicians who have completed the coursework[117]. Minors allowed with second physician's signature.

ID Card

Mandatory.[118] Check the state's health website at www.floridahealth.gov.[119]

Caregivers

No.

Medical Dispensaries

State-licensed dispensaries capped at five stores. The state is working on licensing growers.

---

116 http://www.flsenate.gov/Session/Bill/2014/1030/BillText/er/PDF.

117 http://www.floridahealth.gov/programs-and-services/office-of-compassionate-use/_documents/completed-cme.pdf.

118 http://www.floridahealth.gov/programs-and-services/office-of-compassionate-use/_documents/faq.pdf.

119 http://www.floridahealth.gov/programs-and-services/office-of-compassionate-use/

Georgia Access Rating: Impossible

Medical Law

Georgia HB 1[120] went into effect in 2015, legalized low-THC oil, immunized health care institutions from certain cannabis crimes for dispensing low-THC oil, and created a registry[121] for patients to sign up for protection from arrest for certain cannabis crimes. But you can't legally obtain any products in Georgia.

Qualifying Conditions

Amyotrophic lateral sclerosis, cancer, Crohn's disease, mitochondrial disease, multiple sclerosis, Parkinson's disease, seizure disorder, sickle cell disease.

Limits

Up to 20 ounces of cannabis oil with physician recommendation, but no more than 5 percent THC. Must be labeled. No home-cultivation.

Doctor's Recommendation

Licensed physicians must certify patients to Department of Public Health, with a Certification form.[122] Doctors have to register themselves[123] in the Low THC Registry to certify patients. Finding a licensed physician in Georgia willing to fill out a form may require contacting medical cannabis advocacy groups in Georgia like ProjectCare.[124]

ID Card

Mandatory registration with Department of Public Health Low THC Oil Patient Registry. Fee $25, good for two years. It's called a waiver[125] and you give it to your doctor to file. Patients and caregivers are notified when cards are ready for pickup within 15 business days from a public health office.

Caregivers

Yes, include as patient waiver form.

Medical Dispensaries

No. Residents travel out of state to illegally obtain the drug, and return home with it.

120 http://www.legis.ga.gov/Legislation/en-US/display/20152016/HB/1.

121 http://dph.georgia.gov/low-thc-oil-registry.

122 http://dph.georgia.gov/sites/dph.georgia.gov/files/2015%20Low%20THC%20Oil%20-%20Certification%20Form.pdf.

123 https://sendss.state.ga.us/sendss/!thc.thc_login.

124 http://www.gacareproject.com/.

125 https://dph.georgia.gov/sites/dph.georgia.gov/files/2015%20Low%20THC%20Oil%20-%20Waiver.pdf.

Iowa   Access Rating: Virtually Impossible

Medical Law

Iowa has a CBD law but almost no legal access to the botanical.[126] Forty-six registration cards have been issued, but there's no legal source of CBD in Iowa.[127]

Qualifying Conditions

Intractable seizures.

Limits

Only oral and transdermal forms of CBD allowed. Up to 32 ounces per patient. CBD must come from out-of-state sources.

Doctor's Recommendation

Have your neurologist (or child's neurologist) complete the physician component of the patient application form. Must have undergone at least six months of other unsuccessful treatment.

ID Card

Required. The form to fill out is available for download on the Iowa Health Department's website.[128] Have neurologist and caregiver, if applicable, fill out their portion of the form. Submit completed application, copy of the patient residency documentation, and copies of patient/primary caregiver state-issued driver's license or non-driver identification card to: Iowa Department of Public Health, c/o MCA Registration Card Program, Lucas State Office Building, 321 E. 12th St., Des Moines, IA 50319-0075.

Caregivers

Allowed, 18 and over.

Medical Dispensaries

No.

---

126 http://www.state.ia.us/odcp/docs/CBDFinalFactSheetIowaJune2014.pdf.

127 http://www.idph.state.ia.us/MCARCP/Default.aspx.

128 http://www.idph.iowa.gov

Kentucky Access Rating: Impossible

Medical Law
CBD-only. Signed in 2014. Non-functional. Exempts from the definition of "marijuana" drugs used in FDA-approved studies or compassionate-use programs and the substance cannabidiol when recommended by a physician practicing at a state research hospital.[129] Theoretically, patients in such a trial could get CBD from a Kentucky hemp farm. In practice, nothing is happening.

Qualifying Conditions
Epilepsy.

Limits
As recommended by doctor in a clinical trial.

Doctor's Recommendation
Only theoretically available through clinical trials at the University of Louisville and University of Kentucky research hospitals. In practice, not available.

ID Card
Not available.

Caregivers
No.

Medical Dispensaries
No.

129 http://www.lrc.ky.gov/record/14RS/sb124.htm.

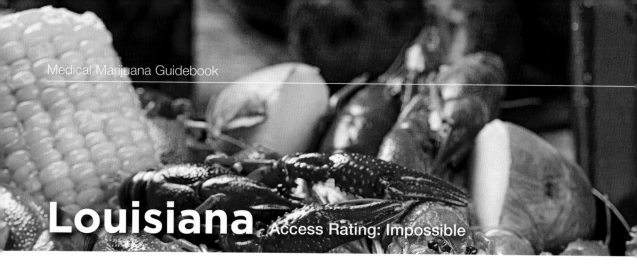

Louisiana Access Rating: Impossible

Medical Law

Louisiana's governor signed the state's first medical CBD law[130] on June 29, 2015, calling for one state-licensed farm and specially licensed pharmacies that will dispense low-THC formulations. The text of law renders it totally impractical. There will be no legal sources of medical cannabis products in Louisiana for several years at least. For more info on what to do, contact groups like the Louisiana Cannabis Association.[131]

Qualifying Conditions

Glaucoma, cancer, quadriplegia.

Limits

Set by physician. Products must have the "lowest acceptable therapeutic levels" of THC possible.

Doctor's Recommendation

Doctors "may prescribe" certain formulations of lowest possible THC formulations "in any form" that are approved by the state's Board of Pharmacy. This is impractical since there are no FDA-approved formulations of cannabis to "prescribe." (Doctors can only "recommend" cannabis to patients.) The Board of Pharmacy will have no formulations to approve — not for several years at least.

ID Card

No card. Your prescription would theoretically be your card.

Caregivers

No.

Medical Dispensaries

Specially licensed pharmacies would theoretically dispense medical cannabis products to patients with a prescription.

---

130 https://www.legis.la.gov/legis/ViewDocument.aspx?d=956617.

131 http://www.louisianacannabis.org/.

Mississippi Access Rating: Impossible

Medical Law
Mississippi has a broken medical cannabis law[132] that gives an affirmative defense to qualified CBD users, of which there are currently none. The "Harper Grace's Law" of 2014 didn't serve a single patient in the state as of 2015.

Qualifying Conditions
Epilepsy.

Limits
CBD oil that is greater than 15 percent CBD and less than .5 percent THC, and obtained from or tested by the National Center for Natural Products Research at the University of Mississippi and dispensed by the Department of Pharmacy Services at the University of Mississippi Medical Center. The university states they are not giving out CBD, and have released no plans[133] to begin doing so.[134]

Doctor's Recommendation
Any doctor can write a recommendation, but document has no legal power because source of legal CBD is not available.

ID Card
No.

Caregivers
No.

Medical Dispensaries
No.

132 http://billstatus.ls.state.ms.us/documents/2014/html/HB/1200-1299/HB1231SG.htm.

133 https://www.umc.edu/news_and_publications/press_release/2014-06-09-00_cannabidiol_oil.aspx.

134 www.umc.edu.

Missouri Access Rating: Very Hard

Medical Law

Missouri is another state that's flunking out of its own medical cannabis program. Missouri passed HB 2238 in 2014[135], legalizing hemp extracts of greater than 5 percent CBD and less than 0.3 percent THC. The state is radically underserving its citizens, but groups like ShowMeCannabis[136] are working to fix the Missouri law.

Qualifying Conditions

Intractable epilepsy.

Limits

Twenty ounces of CBD oil. No home-growing.

Doctor's Recommendation

You have to find one of the rare neurologists in the state with a specialization in cannabinoids to become your doctor, or your child's doctor, and have

them fill out and sign a state Certification Form[137].

ID Card

Patients and their caregivers must get a Hemp Registration Card through completion of an application form[138]. It's thankfully short, just one page. The state has a reported 850 registered CBD patients, but no legal sources.

Caregivers

Only for patient who is a minor.

Medical Dispensaries

Two CBD oil stores are called for but they are not open. The Department of Agriculture[139] is in charge of licensing CBD hemp farms and issued two CBD growing licenses in 2015, reports the state. A scant few patients could see CBD access by 2016.

---

135 http://www.house.mo.gov/billtracking/bills141/sumpdf./HB2238T.pdf.

136 http://show-mecannabis.com/about/.

137 http://health.mo.gov/about/proposedrules/pdf./NeurologistCertificationForm.pdf.

138 http://health.mo.gov/about/proposedrules/pdf./ApplicationForm.pdf.

139 http://agriculture.mo.gov/news/2014/Department_of_Agriculture_Files_Hemp_Production_Rules.

North Carolina Access Rating: Nearly Impossible

Medical Law

Critics call North Carolina's CBD-only medical marijuana law HB 1220[140] of 2014 a "disaster"[141] that's only serving a handful of patients. The North Carolina Epilepsy Alternative Treatment Act removes penalties for doctors who prescribe CBD medications and the patients who take them. It has allowed some small trials of CBD at a few universities.

Qualifying Conditions

Intractable epilepsy.

Limits

Set by neurologist. "Hemp extract" oil must be less than .3 percent THC and greater than 10 percent CBD. No home-cultivation.

Doctor's Recommendation

Neurologist has to be licensed at one of the hospitals in the state, according to proposed new amendments, which passed the Senate in July 2015.[142] The need for "pilot study" enrollment of patients has been dropped. Few North Carolina neurologists have any experience with cannabinoid drugs.

ID Card

The Department of Public Safety is tasked with issuing ID cards to CBD patients, and the cards are not yet available.

Caregivers

Yes, with Registration Card, which is not available.

Medical Dispensaries

No. Three universities (Wake Health, UNC Healthcare, and Duke University Medical Center) are reported[143] to be doing limited trials of CBD drug Epidiolex from GW Pharmaceuticals.

---

140 http://www.ncleg.net/Sessions/2013/Bills/House/PDF./H1220v7.pdf.

141 Bellville, Russ, 2014.

142 http://www.ncleg.net/Sessions/2015/Bills/House/PDF./H766v0.pdf.

143 http://www.wbtv.com/story/28027264/remember-nc-cbd-oils-law-families-say-it-doesnt-work.

Oklahoma Access Rating: Impossible

Medical Law

Signed into law April 2015, Katie and Cayman's Law[144] exempts from marijuana laws certain formulations of CBD, industrial hemp, children in an FDA-approved clinical trial, and adults with a doctor's note for CBD. But there is no CBD legally available in Oklahoma.

Qualifying Conditions

Epilepsy.

Limits

Not more than .3 percent THC in liquid form. No home-cultivation.

Doctor's Recommendation

Get a written certification from a physician licensed in the state to enjoy the exemption.

ID Card

No.

Caregivers

Yes, if parent or guardian.

Medical Dispensaries

No. Patients are bringing CBD and THC in from nearby Colorado.

---

144 http://webserver1.lsb.state.ok.us/cf_pdf./2015-16%20ENR/hB/HB2154%20ENR.PDF.

South Carolina Access Rating: Nearly Impossible

Medical Law

A proposed medical marijuana law in South Carolina failed in 2015, and the state has had a failing CBD-only law, called Julian's Law, since 2014, which legalizes FDA-approved clinical trials of cannabidiol to treat epilepsy patients.[145] Doctors have immunity from arrest for recommending CBD. Qualifying patients with CBD cannot be prosecuted for marijuana crimes. In reality, virtually no one in South Carolina is getting legal CBD. A handful of patients are enrolled in small local clinical trials or in out-of-state trials.

Qualifying Conditions

Dravet syndrome, Lennox-Gastaut syndrome, refractory epilepsy.

Limits

Extracts must contain greater than 15 percent CBD and less than .9 percent THC. No home-cultivation.

Doctor's Recommendation

A document dated and signed by a physician (medical doctor or osteopath).

ID Card

Not available.

Caregivers

No.

Medical Dispensaries

No. Only an approved medical center can give out CBD during a clinical trial, and they have little desire to do so. One trial has been reported[146], at the Medical University of South Carolina, using a CBD oil made by GW Pharmaceuticals.[147]

---

145 http://www.scstatehouse.gov/sess120_2013-2014/bills/1035.htm.

146 http://www.thestate.com/news/business/health-care/article13896149.html.

147 http://www.southcarolinaradionetwork.com/2014/09/03/cannabis-oil-bill-now-law-in-sc-but-families-face-hurdles-for-the-treatment/.

Tennessee
Access Rating: Impossible

Medical Law

Another broken CBD law. Senate Bill 280[148] and SB 2531[149] define "marijuana" to no longer include out-of-state preparations of less than .9 percent THC. Another source of allowed CBD-rich preparations would be a Tennessee doctor running a trial for epilepsy, of which there are virtually none.

Qualifying Conditions

Intractable seizures. Must be part of clinical study.

Limits

No formulations with more than .9 percent THC, and the source of drug must be produced, processed, transferred, dispensed, or possessed by a four-year public institution of higher education "located in any county having a population of not less than seventy-two thousand, three-hundred (72,300) nor more than seventy-two thousand, four-hundred (72,400)." Or a form that "was obtained legally in the United States and outside of this state;

provided that the person shall retain proof of the legal order or recommendation from the issuing state." No home cultivation.

Doctor's Recommendation

Doctors at hospital doing a clinical trial are the only ones who can dispense CBD. Recommending clinicians must be practicing at a hospital or associated clinic, affiliated with an approved university's school of medicine, conducting clinical research on treatment for intractable seizures.

ID Card

No.

Caregivers

No.

Medical Dispensaries

No. CBD must be obtained from a university in Putnam County as part of an approved clinical trial.

---

148 http://www.capitol.tn.gov/Bills/109/Bill/SB0280.pdf.
149 http://state.tn.us/sos/acts/108/pub/pc0936.pdf.

Texas Access Rating: Impossible

Medical Law

A 2015 low-THC law in Texas[150] would, in theory, allow for legal use of CBD products, and calls for a system to manufacture and distribute low-THC cannabis. How it plays out in practice will be another story. The law requires a doctor's "prescription," but since doctors can't "prescribe" cannabis, only recommend it, this law is not functional.

Qualifying Conditions

Epilepsy.

Limits

Formulations of less than .5 percent THC and greater than 10 percent CBD, as "prescribed."

Doctor's Recommendation

The Act calls for a to-be-created registry of doctors who write recommendations, including the dosage prescribed, the means of administration ordered, and the total amount of low-THC cannabis required to fill the patient's "prescription."

ID Card

Mandatory. The Act calls for a to-be-created registry of patients.

Caregivers

No.

Medical Dispensaries

No. The Act calls for dispensing organizations licensed by the state.

---

150 https://legiscan.com/TX/text/SB339/2015.

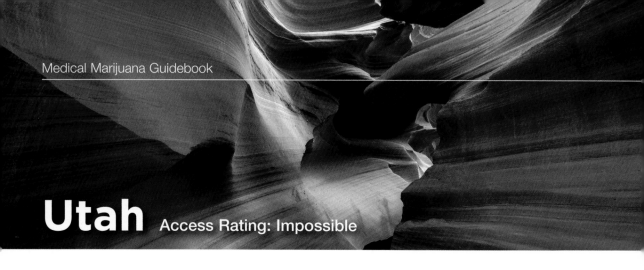

Utah Access Rating: Impossible

Medical Law

The failing medical marijuana state of Utah offers very little to patients besides relatively close proximity to Oregon, Washington, and Colorado. Utah HB 105[151] (Charlee's Law) allows for research hemp farms, exempts patients with intractable epilepsy who possess hemp extract from certain pot crimes, and requires the Department of Health to issue a hemp extract registration card.

Qualifying Conditions

Intractable epilepsy.

Limits

Utah's limits are so lengthy that nothing qualifies in the state. "Hemp extract" must be less than .3 percent THC and at least 15 percent CBD. No home-cultivation. To qualify for exception to the law, CBD oil must originally be obtained as the hemp extract from a sealed container with a label indicating the hemp extract's place of origin, and a number that corresponds with a certificate of analysis; indicates the hemp extract's ingredients, including its percentages of tetrahydrocannabinol and cannabidiol by weight; and is created by a laboratory that is not affiliated with the producer of the hemp extract, and licensed in the state where the hemp extract was produced, and is transmitted by the laboratory to the Department of Health; and that out-of-state CBD provider has a current hemp-extract registration card in Utah.

Doctor's Recommendation

Must be a neurologist and provide written certification, a signed form[152] and an evaluation form[153].

ID Card

Mandatory. Register with the Utah Hemp Registry[154] with an application form[155], fee and neurologist statement. Open to minors with guardian or parent. Mail to: Office of Vital Records and Statistics, Attention: Hemp Extract Registry, P.O. Box 141012, Salt Lake City, UT 84114-1012.

Caregivers

No.

Medical Dispensaries

No. Patients are reportedly bringing in CBD-rich oils from other states, which remains illegal.

151 http://le.utah.gov/~2014/bills/static/hb0105.html.

152 http://health.utah.gov/hempregistry/FINALNCForm052015.pdf.

153 http://health.utah.gov/hempregistry/FINALPE072014.pdf.

154 http://health.utah.gov/hempregistry/index.html.

155 http://health.utah.gov/hempregistry/FINALAPForm052015.pdf.

Virginia Access Rating: Impossible

Medical Law

In 2015, Virginia passed HB 1445[156], which provides an affirmative defense in a prosecution for the possession of marijuana if the marijuana is in the form of cannabidiol oil or THC-A oil, and possessed with a valid written certification from doctor or osteopath. A practitioner shall not be prosecuted for distribution of marijuana under the circumstances outlined in the bill. However, you can't grow CBD-rich cannabis, and stores are illegal.

Qualifying Conditions

Cancer, epilepsy, glaucoma.

Limits

Extracts of at least 15 percent CBD and no more than 5 percent THC.

Doctor's Recommendation

You just need a doctor or osteopath to write you a recommendation to have the affirmative defense.

ID Card

No.

Caregivers

No.

Medical Dispensaries

No. You're going to have to find your own local supplies or import them at your own risk.

---

156 http://leg1.state.va.us/cgi-bin/legp504.exe?151+ful+HB1445+pdf.

Wisconsin Access Rating: Impossible

Medical Law

Wisconsin changed its drug laws in 2014 to exempt CBD[157], and the doctors who recommend it. But there are no legal supplies of CBD in Wisconsin.

Qualifying Conditions

Seizure disorder.

Limits

None.

Doctor's Recommendation

By law, you could get a CBD recommendation from a doctor for a seizure disorder, or a letter or other official documentation stating you possess cannabidiol to treat a seizure disorder.

In reality, cannabinoid-specialized doctors are rare in Wisconsin, and even then, they would have no formulations to recommend that are available in Wisconsin.

ID Card

No.

Caregivers

No.

Medical Dispensaries

No. Theoretically, you could break state and federal law to get CBD oil back into Wisconsin, where you could enjoy an affirmative defense for it. Several dozen Wisconsin residents show up in Oregon's registry data[158].

---

157 https://docs.legis.wisconsin.gov/2013/related/proposals/ab726.

158 https://public.health.oregon.gov/DiseasesConditions/ChronicDisease/MedicalMarijuanaProgram/Documents/ed-materials/ommp_stats_snapshot.pdf.

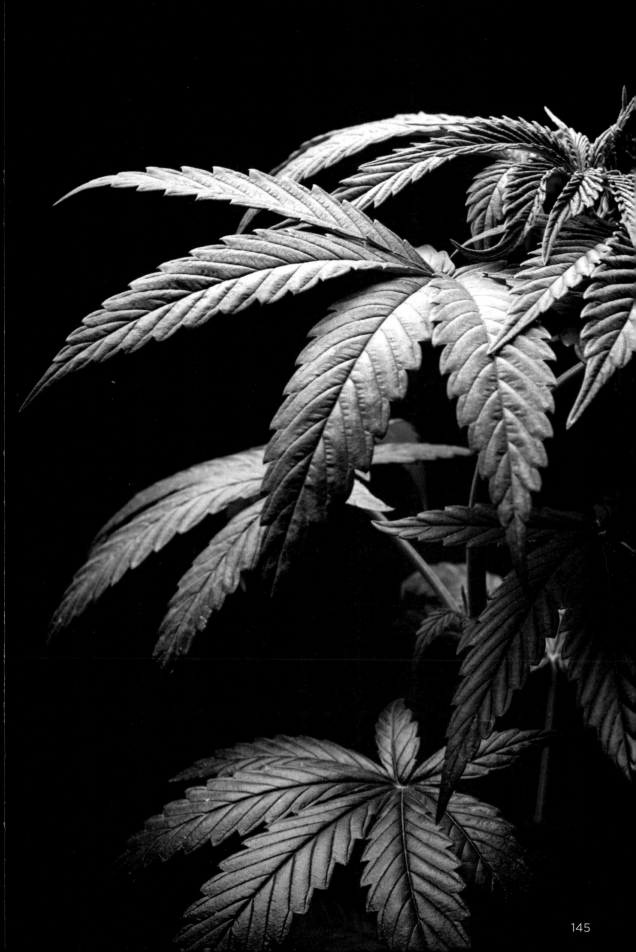

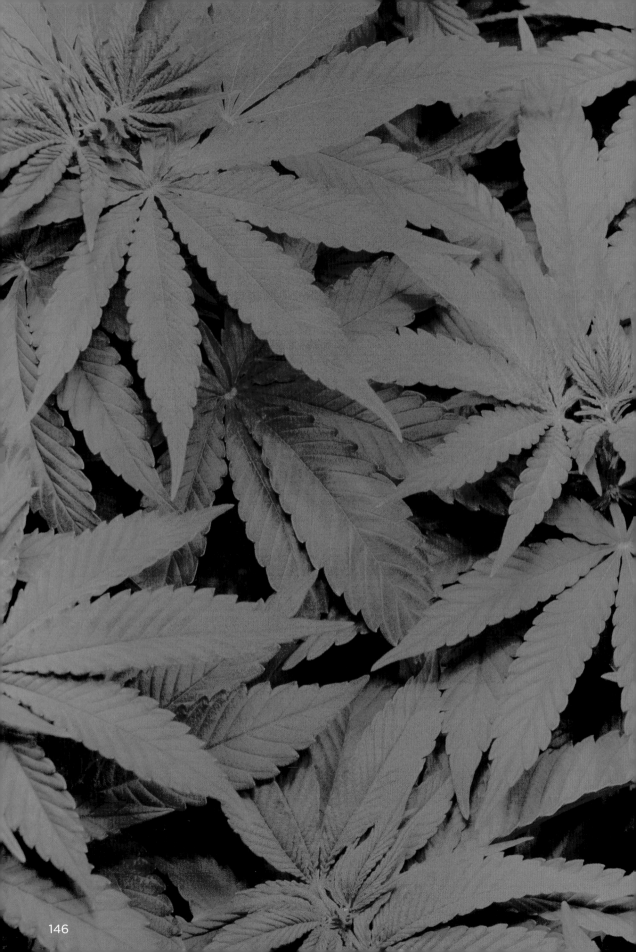

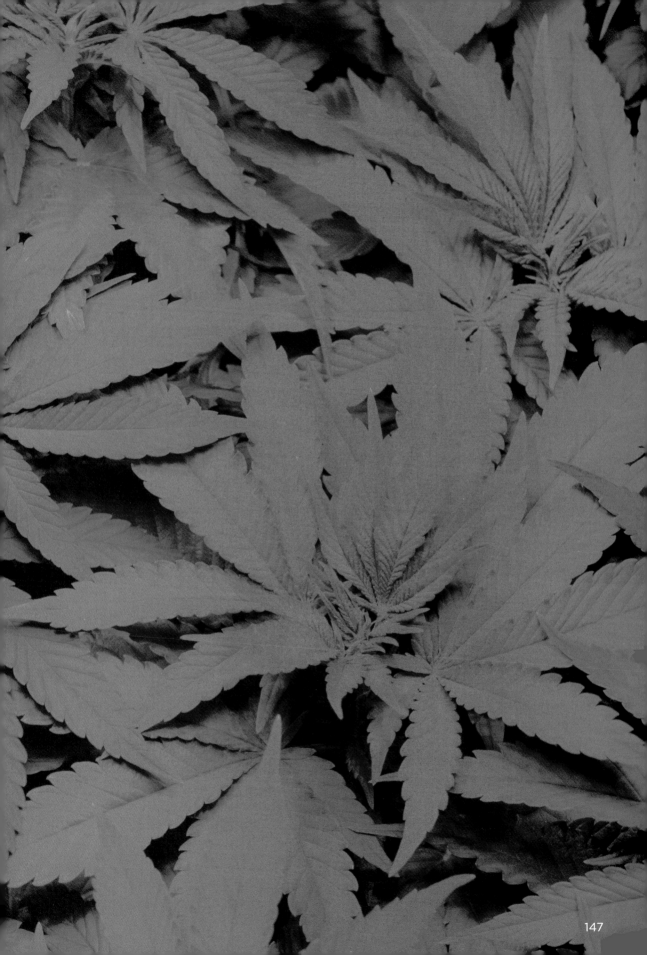

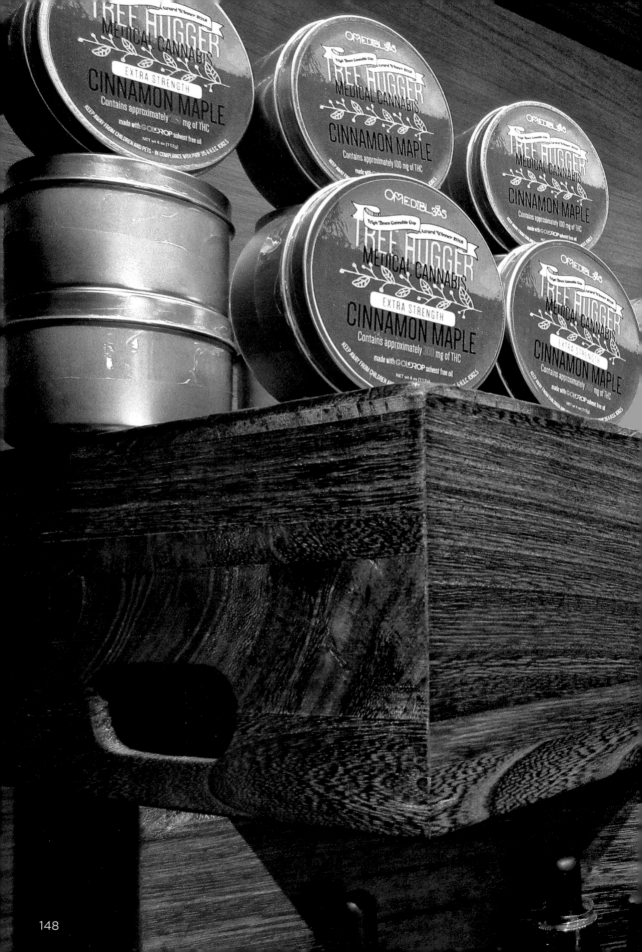

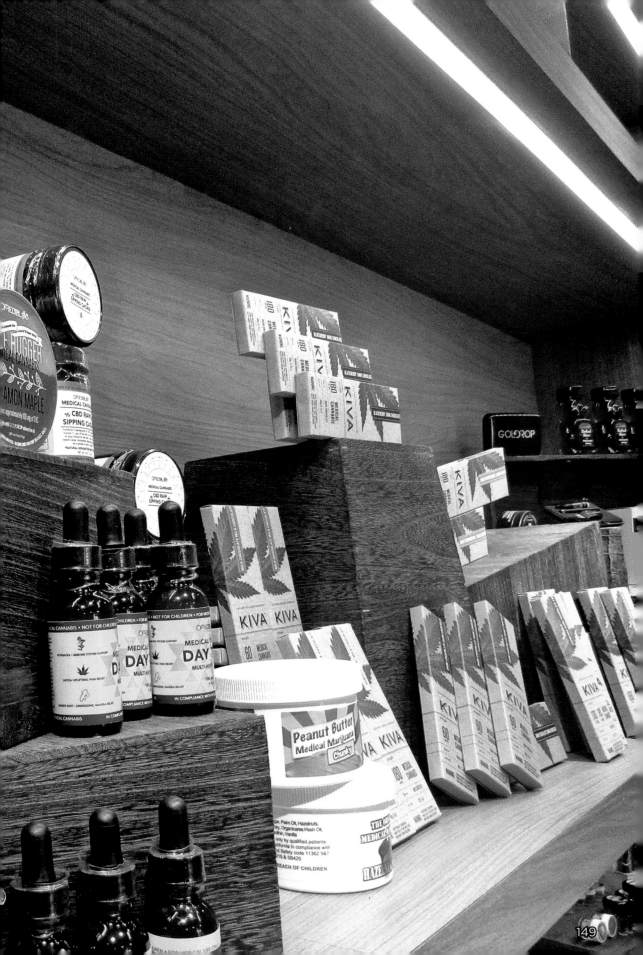

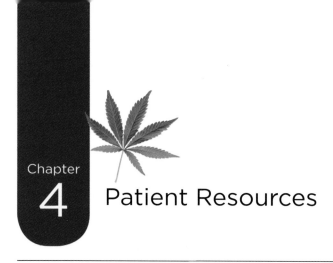

Patient Resources

Finding A Doctor Who Will Recommend Cannabis

Finding a doctor who will recommend cannabis for you can be easy, moderately difficult, hard or impossible, depending on the state you are in and the law's requirements (see Chapter 3 for access rankings and details on your state).

Easy

In states where medical cannabis access is easy, most people use online directories like Yelp.com or WeedMaps.com or others to locate what are often listed as "cannabis clinics." These clinics often advertise in local weekly newspapers as well. Most take drop-in visits, while some might require an appointment. You can expect to pay anywhere from $35 to $100 for such a visit in an easy-access state. The visit is generally not covered by health insurance.

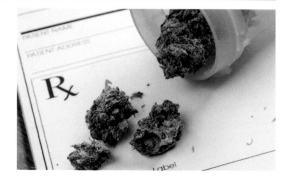

To find a quality specialist, browse the doctor's or clinic's online user reviews and ask other patients for referrals. You are looking for a lot of positive reviews over a long period of time. Visits can take as little as 20 minutes, or if it's crowded, up to an hour.

Be honest with your specialist about why you think you need cannabis. Many patients already use it, and if it's working, tell the specialist. One out of 20 California adults are estimated to have tried medical cannabis (1.4 million people), and 92 percent of them report it worked on a serious condition.[1]

Even in advanced medical cannabis economies, primary care physicians will likely not recommend cannabis, with exceptions for the severely ill — like cancer patients and hospice patients looking for pain relief. Doctors aren't trained on recommending cannabis and they worry about the career repercussions of doing so while inside large health care providers. Generally, the bigger the provider, the less open the institution is to cannabis.

Medium

In states where medical cannabis is harder to access, you might have to drive to another city to find a cannabis-specialized doctor or clinic. Online listings might become more sparse, but they should still exist. Prices might be higher, and visits lengthier and require more medical records.

If you absolutely cannot seem to find a clinician in a medium-access state, contact the state's advocacy organizations for a referral.

Hard

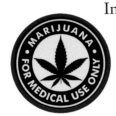

In states where medical cannabis access is hard or impossible to access, doctors who can recommend cannabis will be nearly non-existent. The severely, chronically ill can try begging their primary care physician for a recommendation — you'll never know unless you ask. Patients in these states must contact their state's advocacy organizations for a referral to the few physicians who write recommendations. Mainstream online directories won't have any listings, and if they do, they will be in the state's biggest one or two cities.

Be prepared for lengthy doctor visits. Bring detailed sets of medical records. It can take up to a year to establish a legal doctor-patient relationship in some "hard" states.

Further Doctor Location Resources

The National Organization for the Reform of Marijuana Laws (norml. org) maintains chapters in every state. Contact the chapter through email or social media like Facebook to ask about clinicians.

Americans for Safe Access (safeaccessnow.org) is another national organization dedicated to supporting medical patients, with a presence in each state. Contact your state or region's ASA chapter through listed emails or social media.

There are also many state-level organizations with websites that include doctor directories.

Also, attend medical cannabis-related events like meet-ups, protests, lobby days and festivals to locate clinicians.

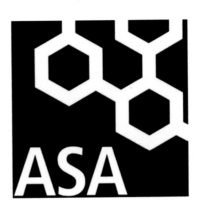

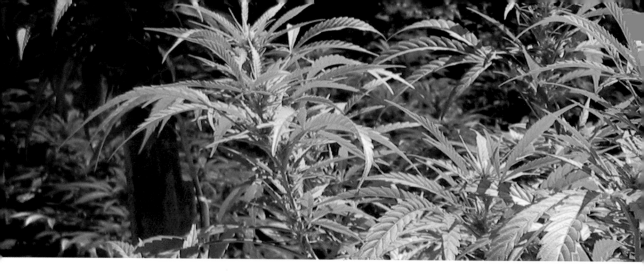

Doctor Education

Doctors who want to become more educated on the endocannabinoid system and medical cannabis can take coursework for Continuing Medical Education credit in certain states.

Contacts:

- Society of Cannabis Clinicians[2], which offers CME credits.[3]

- The International Association of Cannabinoid Medicines.[4]
- TheAnswerPage.com also has an interactive learning series on cannabinoids that offers Continuing Medical Education credit in 15 courses.[5]

Resources for Finding a Caregiver to Assist You

When you're really sick, chances are you're going to need a caregiver to help you obtain medical cannabis.

The most popular caregiver option is a family member like a spouse, or often an adult child or grandchild who is willing to take on responsibility for your care. If the patient is a minor, then his or her parent or guardian will have to be the caregiver. Caregivers often have to be 18 or 21 years old, so check state laws.

If you don't have an immediate family member, extended family member or close friend or acquaintance, you're going to need to get more creative. In advanced medical cannabis economies, many cities have delivery-only collectives that can bring medical cannabis products to your door. They're a great option for elderly, home-bound or hospice patients.

States will often have their own caregivers associations, or you can find them through your state advocacy groups and patient resource centers[6]. Some states like Colorado provide official listings of registered caregivers that are available. Caregivers might also advertise in online listings like Craigslist in certain states.

Good topics to discuss with a potential caregiver include: relevant experience; number of patients they serve; quality of products and how they assure quality; and availability.

Check state laws to make sure your caregiver has a legal amount of patients. Your caregiver might have to register with the state to be legal.

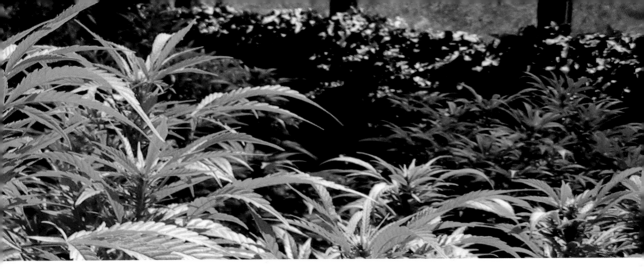

Further Caregiver Location Resources

The American Cannabis Nurses Association[7], Cannabis Patient Network Institute[8], and Patients Out of Time[9] are all great resources for locating a caregiver.

The National Organization for the Reform of Marijuana Laws maintains chapters in each state. Contact your local chapter through email or social media like Facebook to ask about caregivers.

Americans for Safe Access is another national organization dedicated to supporting medical patients, with a presence in each state. Contact your state or region's ASA chapter through email or social media.

Also, attend medical cannabis-related events like meet-ups, protests, lobby days and festivals to locate caregivers.

Finding a Dispensary to Obtain Cannabis

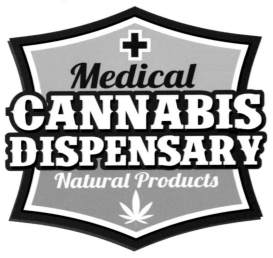

Finding a dispensary can range from being very easy to difficult if not impossible, depending on the state.

In states with high medical cannabis access, dispensaries are plentiful, and you can compare the online reviews of multiple outlets in your area and go check them out. You're looking for well-reviewed, established outlets, preferably some that have won some local awards for products.

You'll always need a valid ID and copy of recommendation to get in the door, and it's generally 18 years and older allowed, with no cell phone use inside.

In easy access states, buying from a dispensary is as easy as finding one, showing up, signing a few forms, having them verify your doctor's recommendation (via phone or web site) and then you buy your cannabis. Most places are cash-only, but most have ATMs on-site.

In medium-access states, you may have to travel to another city to find your nearest dispensary. Again, start

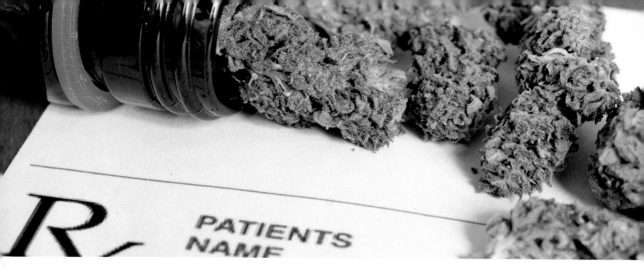

with well-reviewed, established outlets, and work your way down to find the dispensary that's right for you.

In states with very difficult access, you might be have to assign yourself ahead of time to a dispensary, or you might have a choice of one or two in the entire state. In rare cases, you have to make an appointment to visit the dispensary.

Dispensary Directories

The leading site for locating dispensaries is WeedMaps.com, with listings across the United States. WeedMaps tries to list every dispensary, as well as every collective, delivery service and clinician it can find, and those outlets pay WeedMaps for heightened visibility in their directory. Other WeedMaps peers include StickyGuide.com and Leafly.com.

There are also many state-level or local dispensary or delivery directories to be found among the websites of state and regional advocacy or interest groups, and cannabis-focused periodicals like *Culture* magazine, *Cannabis Now*, metropolitan alternative weekly newspapers and some daily newspapers like *The Denver Post*.

Shopping Tips
Buying Flowers

Thoroughly inspect raw cannabis flowers for signs of potency and pathogens. Examine the buds — they should be rich in near-microscopic trichomes, which contain the plant's active ingredients and look like tiny crystals on the surface of the bud. The bud should have no visible contamination like hair, mold or insect feces (which can look like little black specks). Buds can be light to dark green, purple and even red, but flowers should not be brown and overly dry.

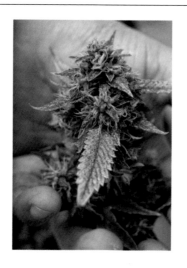

Smell the buds for mold, mildew or anything off. The plant should smell like its terpenes that can resemble thousands of flavors, including skunky, floral or spicy. Trust your reaction to an aroma. Try what smells good. If you can, inspect the bud with your hands. The stem should break with a clean snap and the trichomes should leap into the air like dust.

Ask for and examine the bud's lab test results for THC and CBD, and whether or not it passed tests for mold. Ask if the strain has won any awards or comes with any independent third-party certifications for pesticide-free, organic farming practices. Pesticide use is rampant, even in advanced medical cannabis economies.

Buying Edibles

Be especially cautious buying edibles. Ask for and examine the edibles' lab analysis for THC and CBD, and whether or not it passed tests for mold.

Determine if the source plant for the THC and CBD was an indica or sativa — it could have either sedative or energetic effects.

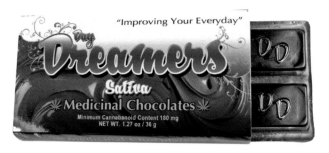

Inspect the edible package. You should see detailed ingredients and nutritional information, as well as dosage and usage instructions. The item should be sealed and tamper-proof, with an expiration date. Ask if the edible has won any awards or comes with any independent third-party certifications for clean kitchen practices.

A test of popular edible products across the nation found potency labeling was wrong much of the time.[10] In a majority of cases, there were less cannabinoids than listed. Weaker-than-expected products often cause patients to react by eating multiple subsequent doses, to ill effect.

Buying Extracts

Be especially cautious buying extracts — they are many times more potent than raw flowers. In many medical states, regulations have not caught up with the rapid rise in the products' popularity.

Ask for and examine the extract's lab test data for THC and CBD, and whether or not it passed residual solvent testing, and if so, what was the parts per million of residual solvent. States are setting residual solvent testing fail limits at anywhere from 50 to 500 ppm.

If the extract was made with ice water, ask to see its tests for mold. Determine if the source plant for the THC and CBD was an indica or sativa, because it can have either sedative or energetic effects.

If the extract comes in the form of an oil for a vape pen, ask what else is in it. Many times, makers cut THC oil with additives to enhance viscosity or flavor. There is almost no research on the healthfulness of inhaling additives like propylene glycol. It's best to avoid them if you can.

Inspect the extract. Generally, lighter extracts are a sign of higher quality, while dark extracts are a red flag. Pure THC-A can be translucent white, light yellow or brown, and any-thing else is the plant's wax, pigment, cell walls or dirt. The extract should be consistent and free of contamination like hair or other debris. Extracts should contain large or trace amounts of the source plant's aroma. Some extracts, especially oils made with carbon dioxide extraction, may not have an aroma. Reject any extracts that smell like chemicals, gas, sulfur or fish. Ask if the extract has won any awards or comes with any independent third-party certifications for safe-source material.

When heated, any sign of accelerated combustion — like sparking or intense flaming — is a red flag for a contaminated extract. A good extract should melt and boil off in clean, consistent vapor, and should smell and taste like its source strain. Stop using an extract if it tastes bad or makes you feel bad.

Growing Your Own Cannabis

If your state allows it, growing cannabis can be a great, cheap and rewarding way to obtain your supply.

Location

Your chief concern will be security and safety. Cannabis plants are a robbery target, with black-market prices running $1,500 per pound of dried outdoor marijuana. One large outdoor plant can yield multiple pounds.

Check for local bans on growing. Preferably, you will grow it in an enclosed, locked, protected outdoor

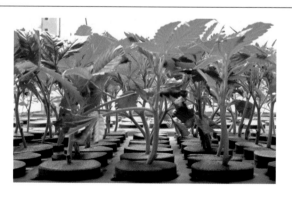

area away from public view or smell — like a greenhouse — or indoors.

Germinating

In states with easy access, you can obtain starting seeds or clones from dispensaries, private collectives or through referrals. Select a strain that will be easy to grow and fits your medical needs.

Cannabis is an annual flowering plant that comes in male and female forms. You can germinate cannabis seeds like many other plants — in a wet paper towel on the counter — then nurture the seedlings in a planting tray. Young plants can be transferred outdoors after the last rain and frost of winter. Indoor grow operations can run year-round.

Vegetating

Under near-constant lights, cannabis will grow bigger. Patients vegetate cannabis in specially amended soil or hydroponic solutions, and have to use water that is the appropriate pH, with the right nutrient levels for the plant. Pest control is a must. Male plants must also be identified and killed, as their pollen ruins a medical crop.

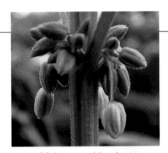

Male cannabis plant.

During its vegetative growth cycle, cannabis prefers a NPK mixture of 10-10-5, and for flowering 5-25-9.

Flowering

Cannabis begins flowering and finishing when it starts receiving anywhere from 8 to 14 hours of uninterrupted darkness each night. Outdoors, this happens in the fall, and depends on latitude and strain. Indoors, growers switch from up to 24 hours of light to about 12 hours on and 12 off. Depending on the strain, cannabis takes eight or more weeks to fully flower. The unfertilized female flower buds become rich in resin and aroma.

Harvesting

For several days before harvest, the plants must be "flushed" — meaning they are fed only water and no nutrients. Flushing allows the plants to use up their store of nutrients so they are not present in the final flowers (Residual nutrients from poor flushing can give buds a more harsh, chemical smell and taste).

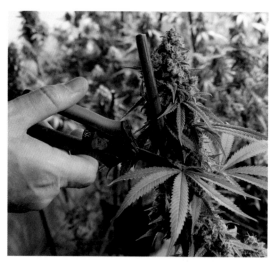

Then the plant is delicately cut down, fan leaves are removed, and branches hung upside down to dry slowly over several days and weeks. Humidity must be kept low and temperature constant to prevent molding

or over-dryness. When the bud's stems can break with a clean snap, the bud is dry enough to be manicured and cured.

Patients or their caregivers trim off all the non-bud leaf and store the buds in airtight Mason jars. They flush the full jars with fresh air first every day, then every few days, then every few weeks. This curing process allows the plant to finish drying. It degrades undesirable ingredients like plant pigment (chlorophyll), and improves taste and smoke immensely.

High-quality cannabis gardening can be an incredibly complex process with a lot of variations. Essential textbooks on how to do it include Ed Rosenthal's *Marijuana Grower's Handbook* and *The Cannabis Encyclopedia* from Jorge Cervantes.

Relocating to a Medical Cannabis State

With access so limited in the United States, and the need so high for this sometimes life-saving medicine, tens of thousands of people are estimated to have begun moving to receive medical cannabis treatment in another state.

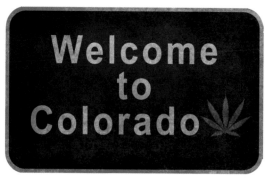

When Do You Know It's Time To Go?

If you live in a hard-to-access medical cannabis state or a CBD state and you are facing a severe, life-threatening illness or condition for which conventional therapies are failing, moving to a different state may be worth it. Some patients are also seeking out medical cannabis as a front-line medicine, as

an alternative to dealing with the potential side effects of conventional pharmaceuticals.

Popular states for medical cannabis refugees are Colorado, because of its proximity to the neediest states in the Midwest, South and East, followed by the western states of California, Oregon and Washington.

Check the local law in your destination state. Many cities ban stores or home-growing.

Moving is very expensive, so many families split up to try medical cannabis in the new state while one member stays at home and earns money. It should be noted that Colorado tends to be more affordable than California or the rest of the West Coast.

You're going to have to tap state patient networks to assist with your relocation, and the Internet and social media is the No. 1 way people do that. For example, the group Pediatric Cannabis Therapy[11] caters to that particular patient set, has thousands of members, and provides online orientation for refugees.

The Facebook group Cannabis Oil Success Stories has 54,000 members who can help refugees with the particulars of moving for care.

Realm of Caring is one of the more prominent refugee advocacy and support groups. It is based in Colorado and has an advanced program of high-CBD product access for those who sign up.[12]

The Undergreen Railroad is an active organization that coordinates fundraising campaigns for medical marijuana refugees.

Americans for Safe Access and NORML chapters and members in each state are helping members with moving.

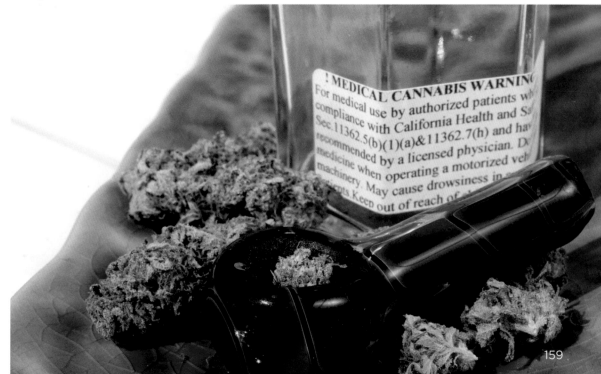

MEDICAL CANNABIS WARNING
For medical use by authorized patients in compliance with California Health and Sa Sec. 11362.5(b)(1)(a)&11362.7(h) and hav recommended by a licensed physician. D medicine when operating a motorized veh machinery. May cause drowsiness in Keep out of reach of

Traveling With Medical Marijuana

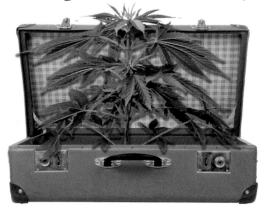

On Foot

About 700,000 Americans are arrested each year in America for marijuana-related crimes, the vast majority of them being simple possession.[13] Travel locally with your medication out of sight. Don't take it out or use it in public, which remains illegal.

Vehicles

Traveling in a vehicle is particularly dangerous with medical cannabis. Never drive while intoxicated on cannabis, and keep all supplies locked in the trunk. Do not volunteer medical cannabis information during a traffic stop. Avoid police encounters by maintaining valid registration and functioning lights, and obeying all traffic laws. In many states, medical cannabis program registration ID cards provide immunity from arrest for certain cannabis crimes.

It is not legal to transport cannabis across state lines, either at the state or federal level. As a practical matter, patients report doing it all the time. Again, you are statistically likely to get arrested for cannabis once every 10 years of daily use.

Bus/Train

Local or regional transportation options often have policies banning cannabis, but they are usually complaint-driven. Make sure to keep pungent flower buds in a smell-proof container. We like DoobTubes for joints and Stink Sacks for raw flowers. Some backpacks now come with carbon filters on them to eliminate smell. Vape pens are great for out-of-the-way use at stops. Amtrak is subject to federal rules.

Air Travel

 Flying with medical cannabis is not legal. It is against federal aviation law to take the medicine on a plane. However, the Transportation Safety Administration has stated that they are not looking for cannabis, and are focused on guns, knives and other weapons or explosives. If they do find cannabis, TSA policy is to turn the contraband over to the local jurisdiction's police department.

Police department policy varies by jurisdiction, and patients report that in states with easy medical cannabis access, they can fly with personal amounts of medical cannabis without a problem. Anything more than a personal amount of medicine is a red flag for drug trafficking. Edibles and extracts can look much more innocuous to security personnel than raw flowers.

Taking medical cannabis out of country violates federal law and the law of the country you are traveling into, which for Americans is mainly Mexico, Canada or Europe. Local restrictions in your tourism destination, especially oversees, may be much more harsh than at home.

Storing Your Medication

Always keep medical cannabis products secure like you would other medications. Use a small, lockable smell-proof case and store it out of sight. Store flowers in a cool, dark place inside an airtight, opaque glass jar to best preserve the bud. Store edibles in a cool, dark place, and if they require refrigeration, in a lockable pouch in the refrigerator or freezer. Thoroughly dispose of edible trash, or your pets may get into it, eat it and suffer an accidental exposure. We like the Stashlogix line of lockable, soft smell-proof bags.[14] A toolbox or gun safe can suffice.

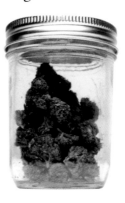

The History of Cannabinoid Science [15 16 17 18 19 20]

The 21st century is fast becoming the century of the endocannabinoid system, and doctors and researchers have only begun to scratch the surface of cannabinoid science. Treatments and cures for dozens of diseases and symptoms are likely to emerge from research into the endocannabinoid system. Indeed, some such medicines are just now coming out.

The main active ingredient in cannabis was discovered long before we had any ideas how it worked inside the human body. But this line of research has vastly broadened our understanding of the human body.

Cannabis' main active ingredient, THC (delta-9-tetrahydrocannabinol), was first isolated and synthesized in a lab in Israel in 1964 by Dr. Raphael Mechoulam, considered the father of cannabinoid science. New sensing techniques including chromotography and nuclear magnetic resonance allowed Mechoulam to isolate specific cannabinoids and test them on monkeys.

Scientists thought THC might work like alcohol, by causing a vast, blanket interference with cell functioning. They were wrong. In 1988, Allyn Howlett, Ph.D, and graduate student William Devane at Virginia Commonwealth University used rat brains and a synthetic cannabinoid tagged with radioactive tritium to figure out how THC docked with mammalian nerve cells. The first distinct cannabinoid receptor (dubbed the CB1) had been located in brain tissue plasma cell membranes.

This discovery is likely on par with the discovery of antibiotics or the dopamine reward system, and researchers like Dr. Mechoulam and Dr. Howlett are considered potential Nobel Laureates for their work.

The existence of a cell receptor system for THC raised the question: "Why do humans have receptors for a plant molecule?" Turns out, we don't. These cell receptors evolved to work with the body's own self-made cannabinoids, dubbed endocannabinoids.

In 1992, a Czech chemist Lumir Ondrej Hanus and William Devane identified the first endocannabinoid, and named it after the Sanskrit word for "supreme bliss" — ananda. They called this endocannabinoid "anandamide," because it also has an "amide" bond. Our body makes anandamide and other endocannabinoids to regulate cell functioning.

In 1993, researchers at Cambridge found a second receptor for the endocannabinoid system, the CB2. In 1995, Dr. Mechoulam and Dr. Sugiura in Japan discovered a second endocannabinoid, dubbed 2-AG.

The race was on to map the body's endocannabinoid system, and scientists located CB1 and CB2 receptors all over the body, and found several more endocannabinoids. The CB1 mostly inhabits the central nervous system, but is also found in body fat, the stomach, placenta, lungs, uterus and liver. CB2 receptors are also all over the body — in the liver, spleen, G-I tract, heart, kidney, bones, endocrine system, lymph and particularly in immune cells. They occur in the peripheral nervous system, but less frequently than the CB1. The ECS plays a role in appetite, blood pressure, brain blood flow, digestion, nausea, immune function, memory, mood, movement, pain, sex, stress and much more. The distribution of receptors explains why cannabis — which has dozens of cannabinoids — has so many indications. As leading research Dr. Ethan Russo said, "Cannabis is the single most versatile herbal remedy on Earth. No other single plant contains as wide a range of medically active herbal constituents."

We now know that the endocannabinoid system constituted a major leap in animal evolution. The evolution occurred roughly 600 million years ago. Everything more evolved than sea sponges — including sea squirts, nematodes and all vertebrate life — has an endocannabinoid system.

With the discovery of the body's endocannabinoid system, its cell receptors and neurotransmitters, scientists have begun to postulate the existence of an endocannabinoid deficiency syndrome to explain a whole host of inexplicable diseases. Researchers theorize that some people are either born with or acquire a dysfunction in their body's own endocannabinoid system. This may include too little or too much anandamide or other endocannabinoid, or an overabundance or lack of cell receptors.

The body's ability to maintain homeostasis is disrupted by this dysfunction, leading to any number of conditions related to the system: mysterious pain, eating disorders, sleep disorders, and other irregularities. Supplementing the system with external doses of cannabinoids like THC and CBD may help such patients, researchers theorize.

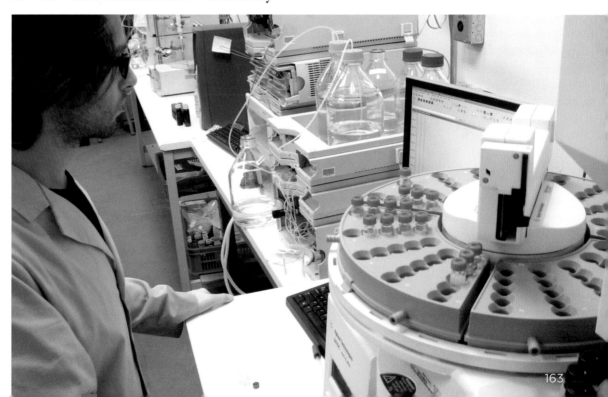

Conversely, humans with a gene mutation leading to statiscally high baseline anandomide levels might be generally happier, less prone to post-traumatic stress, but also more likely to be overweight.

One insight into endocannabinoid system dysfunction comes from the experimental diet drug Rimonabant. THC is widely known to activate the CB1 receptor and encourage appetite. So scientists tried developing a diet drug that would do the opposite: block action at the CB1 receptor to limit appetite. Rimonabant was the result. The synthetic cannabinoid debuted in Europe in 2006 and was found to limit appetite, but the side effects were enormous. Patients reported increased sickness, misery, depression, accidents and suicide. Rimonabant was pulled from the market due to increased risk of suicide.

Further support for endocannabinoid dysfunction syndrome comes from genetically engineered mice. Scientists have made mice without CB1 receptors (CB1 knockout mice) for research purposes, and these are some very miserable mice. CB1 knockout mice show increased anxiety, depression, reduced appetite, weight loss, inability to forget trauma, and increased stress and fear.

Whole plant cannabis therapy still faces research barriers in the U.S. that no other drug on the planet has to deal with. Despite these barriers, scientists are continuing to study individual natural cannabinoids as well as synthetic cannabinoids and their effects on cells, animals and in limited cases, humans. Two whole-plant botanical cannabis formulations are likely to be approved by the FDA for the first time in the coming years, GW Pharmaceuticals' Sativex and Epidiolex, for use in muscle spasticity and epilepsy, respectively.

The American government maintains a monopoly on the only supplies of cannabis approved for research, as well as a bureaucratic blockade on research into any benefits of medical cannabis. But that monopoly and blockade is being challenged and criticized like never before, and the U.S. government is being forced to grow large amounts of cannabis for a new era of human trials.

Furthermore, states with medical cannabis and recreational legalization — as well as other countries — are pushing forward with their own research programs, despite the federal blockade. Pharmaceutical corporations can't patent and profit from a plant like cannabis, so they have little incentive to invest billions of dollars into cannabis' FDA-approval.

However, publicly enacted and taxpayer-supported research programs (like California's Center for Medicinal Cannabis Research[21] and Colorado's Department of Public Health[22] research grants, and the University of Washington[23]) offer some of the best hope for botanical cannabis science without the bias of the federal government's war on drugs.

The History of Cannabis & Its Prohibition

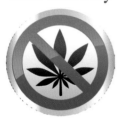

Very few people understand the history of cannabis, or any plants for that matter, but that history explains America's medical cannabis access problem. We have large amounts of evidence that cannabis has been used by humans for at least 10,000 years[24] in every habitable continent for a wide variety of purposes, including food, fuel, fiber and medicine.

Cannabis is so versatile, each society has found the need to place laws on the plant, sometimes mandating it be grown for hemp purposes, as in the early United States, other times banning and demonizing it. In Western civilization, cannabis prohibition can be traced to the Spanish Inquisition.

Evolution

According to ancient pollen analysis, cannabis evolved out of the nettles family of plants tens of millions of years ago in what we now call central Asia. And today it inhabits a plant family that includes hops and several species of hackberry. The cannabis genome also split due to eons-long geographical changes in Asia into a more fiber-producing variety (very low in THC), and a more psychoactive drug plant variety (high in THC). Like other plants, cannabis evolved to secrete oily resins to deter pests and predators. THC may also protect plants from sun damage, as it blocks UV radiation.

Domestication

Cannabis is a fast-growing weed that does well in places cleared by early humans, and humans first began using cannabis in central Asia. It has some of the strongest fibers in nature, and its plentiful seeds are rich in fatty, nutritious oils. Early man quickly recognized cannabis for its medicinal properties and it's been part of written medical textbooks since about 1500 B.C.[25]

Global Spread

Humans spread cannabis throughout the ancient world, and it was used by medieval pharmacists in tincture form. Hemp was also a massive crop for medieval Europe.

New World

To the best of our knowledge, the Spanish brought cannabis to the New World in the form of the hemp rigging that held together their ships. The

Spanish Crown mandated hemp be sown in the New World. Indigenous people were master herbalists and quickly added the drug to their advanced selection of botanical drugs.[26]

Medical cannabis tincture was available in pharmacies in the United States, Europe and Mexico at the time "marijuana" began being prohibited — first in Mexico in 1920. Lurid tales of marijuana madness among the lower class traveled north along the first news wire services, leading to pre-emptive bans on marijuana in certain states. Colorado and California were among the first states to prohibit marijuana, though legislators rarely knew specifically what they were prohibiting. Medical cannabis tincture remained available on pharmacy shelves.

Prohibition

With several dozen states prohibiting marijuana, anti-narcotics officials worked to pass a blanket federal prohibition, in the form of a tax too high for anyone to pay. The American Medical Association was one of the most ardent defenders of medical cannabis in Congress. An AMA representative said cannabis was a vital, if variable, part of a physician's toolkit. But cannabis prohibition swept in amid a wave of New Deal-era government programs that would also lead to failed alcohol prohibition from 1920-1933.[27]

American ambassadors tried to take cannabis prohibition global with the first international narcotics treaties, beginning in the 1910s. The U.S. also erected layers of barriers to prevent medical researchers from ever being able to study the plant.

In 1967, President Richard Nixon declared an all-out war on marijuana as a pretext for targeting opposition and protest groups. Nixon overruled the findings of his own hand-picked National Commission on Marihuana and Drug Abuse, which called for decriminalization.

The wave of recreational cannabis legalization support ebbed through the 1970s, and in its place came the "Just Say No" era under President Ronald Reagan. Marijuana had become a symbol in a much larger culture war between progressives and conservatives, coastal states and the center of the country, whites and minorities, and the affluent versus the poor.

Marijuana became the most common drug arrest, and drug arrests became the most common type of arrest in the country.[28] Marijuana prohibition fell disproportionately on the poor and people of color. America became the world leader in incarceration rates per capita, and blacks became 3.73 times as likely to be arrested for pot than whites, despite similar usage patterns.

Still, usage levels remained stubbornly unchanged.

Medical Marijuana

By the mid-90s, activists were ready for a new tack. Polls consistently showed folks were using medical marijuana, and that it worked, and they supported the medical use of it. Voters passed the Compassionate Use Act in California in 1996, setting off a global debate that has led to 23 states with medical cannabis laws.

While studying the benefits of whole plant cannabis is not permitted by law, researchers analyzed the plant's individual molecules and how they worked in animals and humans — building a massive archive of evidence supporting the plant's medical efficacy.

Today, 78 percent of Americans support lawful access to medical cannabis.[29][30]

In 2014, Congress passed a historic cease-fire in the war on medical marijuana in America: No Department of Justice funds can be spent interfering with state medical marijuana laws. The bipartisan measure was just the beginning of a series of ongoing measures to unwind the war on marijuana, and end the blockade on its research.

This is a legal medical document, and its purpose is solely to affirm that the use of cannabis (marijuana) for medical purposes may be appropriate for the patient listed above. This document is to be used to help law enforcement officers identify individuals whose possession and cultivation of medical cannabis (marijuana) is legal and permissible pursuant to Health and Safety Code Section 11362.5 and SB420.

I have evaluated the medical risks and benefits of cannabis use with the patient. I recommend/approve of my patient's use of medical marijuana as it pertains to their current condition...

This letter qualifies my patient for...

_____ One month _____ Three months _____ Six months _____ One year

of medical cannabis usage, unless otherwise noted. This recommendation

Today's Date - MAR 1 6 2012   Expires on ___ MAR 1 6 2013

Cannabis & the Limits of the Law

Medical cannabis prohibition in America is a multi-layered policy, with plenty of pitfalls that can hurt a patient's life and well-being. The plant remains federally illegal, and while practically no patients are arrested on federal pot possession charges, providers are. State law application is uneven, especially in more conservative, recalcitrant counties. Patients also encounter a patchwork of local regulations.

Moreover, medical cannabis patients can still lose their job, house, kids, or even an awaited organ transplant — all for otherwise lawful medical cannabis use.

Under the Controlled Substances Act of 1970, marijuana is a federally illegal Schedule 1 drug, considered as dangerous as heroin or LSD. According to arrest statistics, the vast majority of marijuana arrests are made by local and state officials. Each state has its own drug laws, and they often overlap with the federal government's laws. In the case of medical cannabis, the laws are diverging. State laws often provide a shield in state court (affirmative defense), or straight-up legalize certain activity for cardholders. The limited CBD-only states often exempt CBD from their state's definition of "marijuana."

So, in practical application, the federal drug war is a state drug war, and patients should generally be more focused on what is legal in their state. A recent White House memo also told federal prosecutors to focus on armed, interstate drug trafficking cartels, and not licensed, controlled state cannabis distribution systems or patients.

Among state systems, the principle of "local control" reigns supreme. Cities and counties often have the power to ban recreational cannabis stores or medical dispensaries, or even the cultivation of a single plant. Local control allows America to be flexible enough to accommodate deeply conservative areas biased against cannabis, and those that want to access to it. The downside is patients face a patchwork of rules in each state that are constantly shifting as America evolves on cannabis. Local ordinances are where cannabis law has its biggest impact, and it's imperative patients stay abreast of local rules through their state advocacy organizations and its local chapters.

Employment

Most states allow employers to fire employees for lawfully using medical cannabis in their off hours, even if they have never been intoxicated at work. A few states have employment protections. Groups like ASA are working to create workplace anti-discrimination in every state. You can get fired for failing a drug test for marijuana, even if you are a lawful patient. Hide your patient status at work, and avoid using cannabis for 30 days before a urinalysis screening.

Education

Generally, schools and universities do not have to accommodate lawful cannabis use. Students can lose student aid over a marijuana misdemeanor. On-campus use is routinely barred. Educators who use medical cannabis may face reprisals, depending on school policy. Very few states have anti-education discrimination policies for patients, especially pediatric patients.

Health Care

Many states allow hospitals and doctors to discriminate against medical cannabis patients when it comes to treating them, or prescribing drugs, and organ transplants. Patients might have to change doctors and leave a large provider for a more knowledgeable specialist in their area. Patients are routinely asked to discontinue lawful medical cannabis use or lose their prescriptions for other drugs like opioids. Informing your life insurance provider of medical cannabis use may cause your rates to rise, sometimes dramatically.

Parenting

Child welfare authorities are interested in the health and safety of children, and in their eyes, a parent who uses cannabis is akin to one who uses heroin or LSD: a potential danger to the health and safety of a child. Pregnant, birthing and nursing moms who test positive for THC can and do trigger Child Protective Services investigations. Parents who lawfully use medical cannabis can lose their children in CPS investigations — especially if a child is accidentally exposed to THC if the medicine is left out. Home-growing is also seen as a potential risk to the

> If you're in the presence of children, it's generally a bad idea to be consuming cannabis. If in strictly adult company, it's polite to ask before smoking or vaping. Sometimes the discretion offered by tinctures and edibles can really come in handy. If you're alone, who's gonna stop you?

health and safety of the child — due to any potential for robbery, or exposure of the child to the plants, any loose wiring, and the potential for mold during indoor growing. Getting your kids back can take months and large amounts of money in legal fees, and patients may be asked to test clean of THC and take mandatory drug classes to get their kids back.

Medical cannabis use can also become an issue in divorce proceedings. Parents can lose custody or visitation rights for medical cannabis use, in certain circumstances.

Parole/Probation

Patients on parole or probation can be re-arrested and re-imprisoned for otherwise lawful medical cannabis use, if not using THC is a condition of their probation or parole.

In all these ways and many more, medical cannabis patients are very much second-class citizens in the United States. We urge patients and their allies to work actively with state advocacy groups to change such laws before they ever affect you or a loved one. If you need a lawyer, a good resource for a criminal defense attorney licensed in your state is the NORML legal database[31].

Does Cannabis Cure Cancer?

Maybe, in some cases. Using cannabis certainly doesn't appear to hurt most cancer patients receiving conventional treatment.

We have a lot of reliable cell, culture and some animal studies showing cannabinoids treat some types of cancers in mice and rats.

There is a lot of anecdotal evidence that high doses of cannabinoids, especially THC, can cause remissions of cancer, but the evidence is pretty poor, and far from conclusive. One study of intravenous THC in patients with untreatable brain cancer showed it helped some and didn't hurt anyone. Doctors in Israel who looked at a large sample of cancer patients found those on cannabis had a higher quality of life, but did not live longer.

Due to federal drug research barriers, cannabinoids for cancer is an incredibly difficult research field to work in, and we need exhaustive clinical studies to determine how to best use cannabinoids on cancer.[32]

For use of cannabis as a complimentary and alternative medicine, check out Dr. Donald Abrams' textbook Integrative Oncology.[33]

Further Legal Information Resources Online

Americans for Safe Access

Americans for Safe Access (safeaccessnow.org) has emerged as one of the chief medical marijuana patient advocacy organizations in the United States. Their website lists generally recent medical marijuana laws, broken down by state, and they publish a number of patient resources.

NORML

The National Organization for the Reform of Marijuana Laws is one of the nation's oldest, most stalwart advocates for adult-use legalization, and by extension, legal medical marijuana. Their website, norml.org, also aggregates state laws, has directories and provides news.

The National Conferences of State Legislatures

This group represents the interest of the individual states at the federal level. In 2015, the NCLA passed a resolution asking the federal government to respect state marijuana laws, and the NCLS tracks state laws.[34]

Further Health & Science Resources Online

PubMed

A central repository for medical research, PubMed allows public searches in its database, yielding thousands of abstracts from cannabis-related studies.

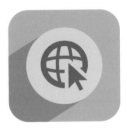

NCI PDQ CAM

The National Cancer Institute's Physician Data Query Complimentary and Alternative Medicines listing for cannabis summarizes existing medical research on the use of cannabis and cannabinoids for the treatment of cancer. It's among the most professionally vetted sources of information for physicians.[35]

Project CBD

Project CBD has led the country in publicizing research into the medical uses of cannabidiol (CBD) and other cannabinoids. The site summarizes CBD science and provides news, directories and other resources.[36]

International Association for Cannabinoid Medicines

A medical resource for cannabinoid researchers and others who are interested, the International Association for Cannabinoid Medicines website hosts Q/As, current studies, medical uses of cannabinoids, side effects and definitions, and you can subscribe to the IACM bulletin.

ClinicalTrials.gov

Patients can join clinical trials of cannabis and cannabinoids by reviewing trials and applying through Clinical-Trials.gov.[37] More than 200 trials related to marijuana were listed in 2015.

A Guide to Activism Resources Online

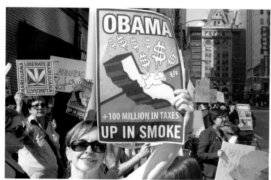

Being a medical cannabis patient means staying engaged in local, regional, state and national politics to protect your rights and work to end ongoing discrimination.

Marijuana Policy Project

With the slogan "We change laws" the Marijuana Policy Project (mpp.org) is among the most effective drivers of pot policy reform in America. It has been the force behind a number of winning state-level ballot initiatives (including Colorado's historic Amendment 64), as well as legislative bills. MPP also fields lobbyists in Congress who are making unprecedented strides toward winding down the federal war on marijuana.

Americans for Safe Access

America ns for Safe Access (safeaccessnow.org) advocates for medical cannabis patients statewide in a number of ways, including lobbying Congress. Join ASA to stay abreast of national changes, and take action at the local level. In 2015, ASA succeeded in ending organ transplant discrimination against qualified patients in California, among other victories.

Drug Policy Alliance

The Drug Policy Alliance (drugpolicy.org) helped fund the first medical marijuana legalization initiative in California in 1996, and has been among the most active agents for change across the spectrum of drug law reforms ever since. The DPA is working at the state level to tax and regulate cannabis for adult use in California in 2016 — which will broaden access for medical patients. The DPA also fields Congressional lobbyists working to end America's incarceration epidemic.

American Civil Liberties Union

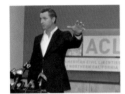

The ACLU (aclu.org) has emerged in the last few years as among the most credible advocates for protecting state-legal medical cannabis patients and promoting adult-use legalization as a means to the end of the drug war. The ACLU ran Washington's winning initiative in 2012, and has released a series of bombshell reports highlighting the disparities in marijuana enforcement amongst blacks and whites.

The National Organization for the Reform of Marijuana Laws

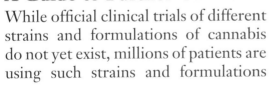

Around since the 1970s, NORML (norml.org) is one of the nation's oldest advocates for cannabis users' rights. With chapters in nearly every state and major city, NORML remains a hub for activists in the modern era.

A Guide to Further Online Advice and Information

While official clinical trials of different strains and formulations of cannabis do not yet exist, millions of patients are using such strains and formulations and reporting back their findings using a wide variety of online methods.

Leafly

Leafly.com is one of the Internet's most prominent locations to look up different strains and learn about their genetics, and reported effects. The site includes copious amounts of user reviews about different strains. The reviews are of varying quality, but can help inform patients' strain choices.

StickyGuide

StickyGuide.com is another leading Internet resources for dispensary menus that also lists products by indication, such as "pain" or "insomnia." StickyGuide users can search their area based on indication to find products that might be right for them.

Seedfinder

Cannabis is a global, multi-billion industry where lots of money is riding on particular new strains, their purported effects and patient reviews. As such, the cannabis seed directory Seedfinder can be a useful resource for patients looking to learn more about a strain. Growers often list information on strain effects and indications. The information is not independent, third-party information, but a grower's reputation is everything, so there is a profit motive for developing great new strains and advertising factually (http://en.seedfinder.eu/).

Online Forums

Millions of medical marijuana patients are discussing products like never before using a variety of online forums like those found at www.420magazine.com/forums and elsewhere. Popular online forums include patients discussing which strain and product they use for particular indications. Other large, active forums include grasscity.com and cannabisculture.com. Also, activist "Granny Storm Crow" has compiled one of the Internet's biggest repositories of links to cannabis research, by indication, available at grannystormcrowslist2014.webs.com.

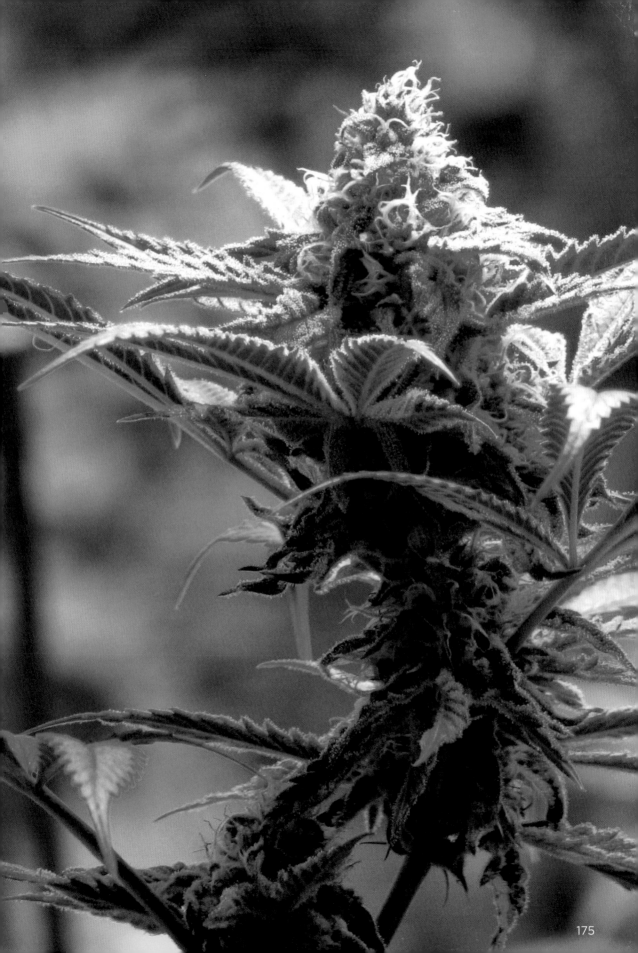

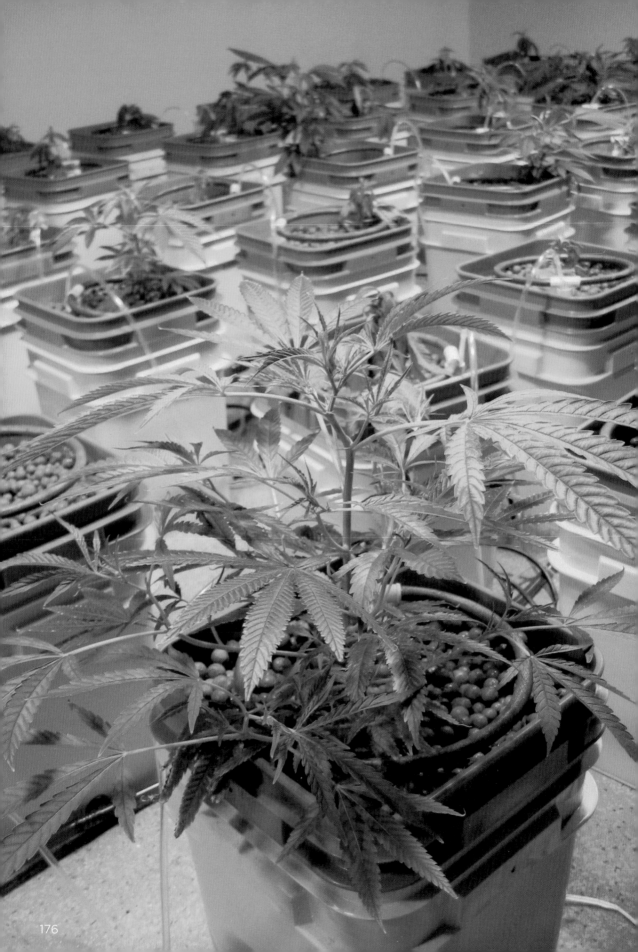

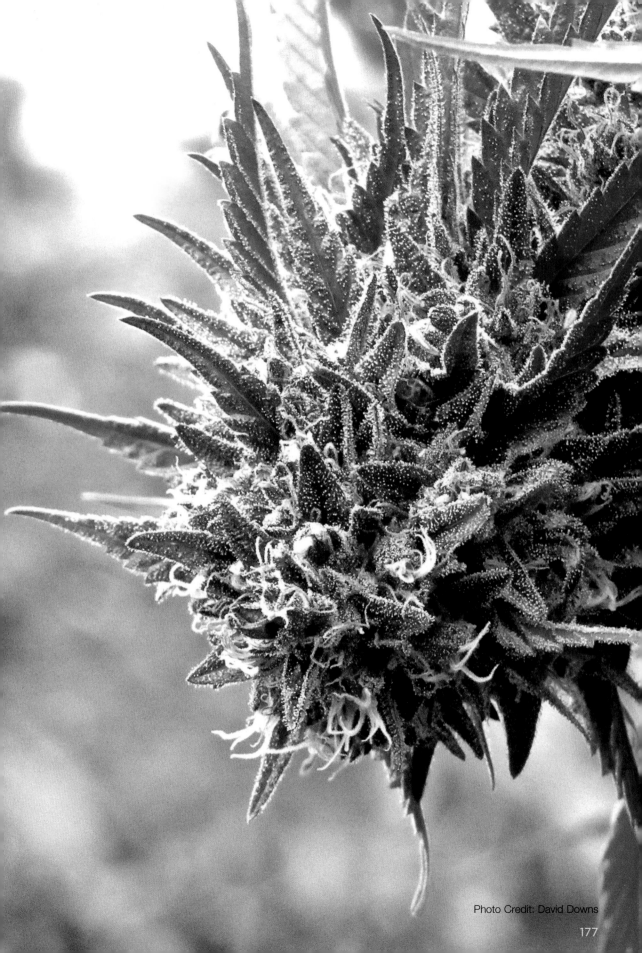

Photo Credit: David Downs

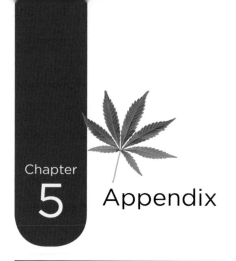

Suggested Reading

Cannabis Pharmacy: The Practical Guide to Medical Marijuana (Black Dog & Leventhal, 2014). Michael Backes has penned one of the most practical books on medical cannabis use in America based on his extensive experience serving patients as well as working with Project CBD, the International Association for Cannabinoid Medicines, and the American Herbal Products Association's Cannabis Committee.

Handbook of Cannabis (Oxford University Press, 2014). Edited by leading researcher Roger G. Pertwee, this massive, 768-page compendium covers the history of cannabis, and its legal and heath issues.

Cannabis (Reaktion Books, 2014). Part of Reaktion Press' series of books on different plants, author Chris Duvall focuses on the plant's evolution and geography, as well as the origins of its names and confusion over its properties. It's extremely scholarly and current.

The Pot Book: A Complete Guide to Cannabis (Park Street Press, 2010). Dr. Julie Holland, M.D., edits this collection on cannabis' medical uses, potential, politics and history, with contributions from Andrew Weil, Michael Pollan, Lester Grinspoon, Rick Doblin, Ph.D., and Raphael Mechoulam.

Stoned: A Doctor's Case for Medical Marijuana (2015). David Cassarett, M.D.'s personal journey into accepting medical cannabis as a physician parallels the story of Dr. Sanjay Gupta, who when confronted with the facts and the patients, emphatically began supporting cannabis therapies.

Marijuana Legalization: What Everyone Needs to Know (Oxford University Press, 2012). Researchers at the RAND Drug Policy Research Center tackle the most salient questions about marijuana in a breezy, question-and-answer format. It's a great reference for baseline data on America's use of cannabis.

Marijuana, Gateway to Health (Dachstar Press, 2011). Researcher activist Clint Werner turns cannabis dogma on its head with a thoroughly researched meta-analysis of the benefits of cannabis. Also includes a short history of the medical marijuana movement.

Ed Rosenthal's Marijuana Grower's Handbook (Quick American, 2010). One of two of the canonical guides to growing cannabis at home, this book is 510 pages, covering everything from selecting seeds to storing your finished crop.

The Cannabis Encyclopedia (Van Patten Publishing, 2015). Lifelong cultivator and former *High Times* cultivation editor Jorge Cervantes just completed his updated *The Cannabis Encyclopedia* — a masterwork on how to grow cannabis that is 596 pages.

The Official High Times Cannabis Cookbook (Chronicle Books, 2012). Veteran *High Times* staffer Elise McDonough put together this lushly illustrated 160-page guide to safely making and eating your own cannabis-infused recipes. Comes with easy-to-follow recipes for infusing butter and other oils with cannabis, and then offers dozens of delicious recipes.

Big Book of Buds Vol. 1 - 4 (Quick American, 2011). Celebrity cultivation author Ed Rosenthal aggregates photos and strain information from the world's best breeders, which can provide valuable insights into strain uses.

Beyond Buds (Quick American, 2014). Vaporizers and extracts are the focus of this "how-to" book, which covers the major types of vaporizers and extracts and how they work, as well as how to make extracts like tincture on your own.

Home Grown (UNC Press, 2014). Historian Isaac Campos dives deep into the origin of American cannabis prohibition — in Mexico. This heavily researched, riveting history book helps illuminate how cannabis went from ancient medicine, to the Mexican scourge of "marijuana."

The Protectors: Henry J. Anslinger and the Federal Bureau of Narcotics 1930-1962 (University of Delaware Press, 1990). The late historian John C. Williams' out-of-print book is an essential historical analysis of the rise of cannabis prohibition in America, illustrating how the misunderstood plant got swept up in much larger historical forces like the New Deal and international treaty politics.

Smoke Signals: A Social History of Marijuana - Medical, Recreational and Scientific (Scribner, 2013). Writer/researcher Martin Lee's 568-page "social history" spans 2,700 years, with an emphasis on explaining how cannabis came to be prohibited in the U.S.

Cannabinoids [38, 39]

Below is a list of the main active cannabinoids and their medical effects:

Δ-9-tetrahydrocannabinol (THC) — CB1 agonist, euphoriant, analgesic, anti-inflammatory, antioxidant, anti-emetic, bronchodilator, muscle relaxant.

cannabidiol (CBD) — anxiolytic, analgesic, antipsychotic, anti-inflammatory, antioxidant, anti-spasmodic, treatment of addiction, anti-diabetic, antiemetic, neuroprotectant, anti-psychotic.

cannabinol (CBN) — Oxidation breakdown product, sedative, antibiotic, effective against MRSA, analgesic, anti-spasmodic, anti-inflammatory, antioxidant.

cannabichromene (CBC) — anti-inflammatory, antibiotic, anti-fungal, anti-depressant in rodent model, bone stimulant.

cannabigerol (CBG) — anti-inflammatory, antibiotic, anti-fungal, anti-depressant rodent model, effective against MRSA, bone stimulant.

tetrahydrocannabivarin (THCV) — CB1 agonist, analgesic, euphoriant, anorectic (suppresses appetite), anti-convulsant, bone stimulant.

Δ-9-tetrahydrocannabinol acid (THC-A) — anti-proliferative, anti-spasmodic.

Terpenes [40]

Below is a list of the some of the main smell and flavor molecules in cannabis, and their reported medical effects.[41]:

myrcene — analgesic, anti-inflammatory, antibiotic, anti-mutagenic, sedating, muscle relaxant, hypnotic.

caryophyllene — anti-inflammatory, cytoprotective, (gastric mucosa), anti-malarial.

d-limonene — cannabinoid agonist, immune potentiator, antidepressant, antimutagenic, anxiolytic, causes breast cancer cells to commit suicide, kills acne bacteria, treats gastric reflux.

linalool — sedative, antidepressant, anxiolytic, immune potentiator, local anesthetic, anticonvulsant.

pulegone — AChE inhibitor, sedative, antipyretic.

1,8-cineole (eucalyptol) — AChE inhibitor, Increases cerebral blood flow, stimulant, antibiotic, antiviral, anti-inflammatory, antinociceptive.

pinene — anti-inflammatory, bronchodilator, stimulant antibiotic, anti-neoplastic, AChE inhibitor.

terpineol — sedative, antibiotic, AChE inhibitor, antioxidant, anti-malarial.

terpineol-4-ol — AChE inhibitor, antibiotic.

Nerolidol — sedative, skin penetrant, anti-malarial.

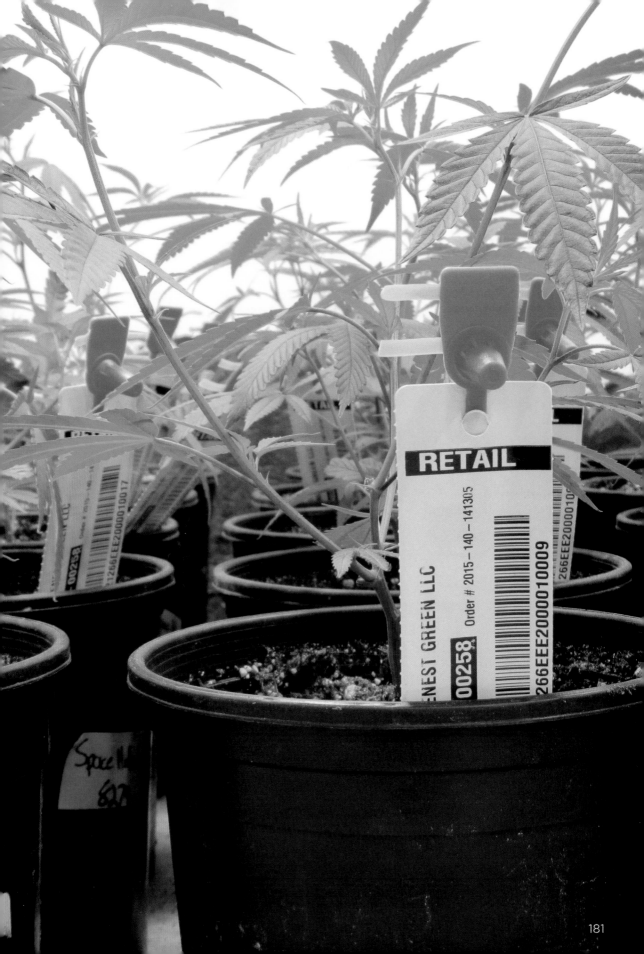

RETAIL

00258 Order # 2015 – 140 – 141305

ENEST GREEN LLC

266EEE2000010009

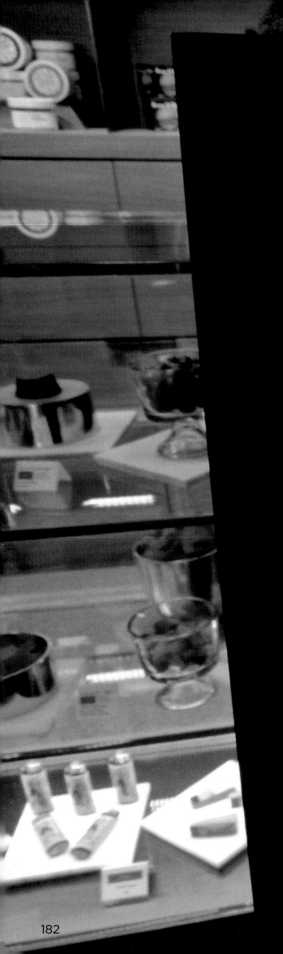
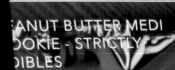

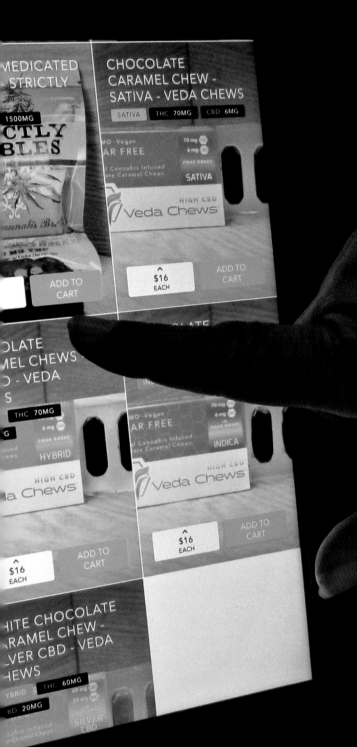

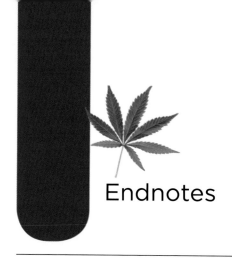

Endnotes

Disclaimer

Nothing in this book is meant to treat any symptom or disease. Only a licensed physician, naturopath, osteopath or registered nurse who is specialized in cannabis can tell you if the botanical is right for you, and fully explain its risks and side effects.

Endnotes

1 Survey

2 http://cannabisclinicians.org/

3 http://cannabisclinicians.org/medical-cannabis-continuing-education-cme-course/

4 http://cannabis-med.org/

5 http://theanswerpage.com/library.php?sid=8

6 http://mmmpcaregiverfinder.org/

7 http://www.americancannabisnursesassociation.org/

8 http://www.cpninstitute.org/

9 http://www.medicalcannabis.com/

10 Vandrey R, Raber JC, Raber ME, Douglass B, Miller C, Bonn-Miller MO. Cannabinoid Dose and Label Accuracy in Edible Medical Cannabis Products. JAMA. 2015;313(24):2491-2493. doi:10.1001/jama.2015.6613.

11 http://pediatriccannabistherapy.com/

12 https://www.theroc.us/

13 FBI, 2014

14 http://www.stashlogix.com/

15 Russo EB. History of cannabis and its preparations in saga, science, and sobriquet. Chem Biodivers. 2007 Aug;4(8):1614-48. PubMed PMID: 17712811.

16 Pertwee RG. Pharmacological actions of cannabinoids. Handb Exp Pharmacol. 2005;(168):1-51. Review. PubMed PMID: 16596770.

17 Fine PG, Rosenfeld MJ. The endocannabinoid system, cannabinoids, and pain. Rambam Maimonides Med J. 2013 Oct 29;4(4):e0022. doi: 10.5041/RMMJ.10129. eCollection 2013. PubMed PMID: 24228165; PubMed Central PMCID: PMC3820295.

18 Werner, Marijuana Gateway to Health +w, 2011

19 Backes, Cannabis Pharmacy, 2014

20 Pertwee, editor, Handbook of Cannabis, 2014

21 http://www.cmcr.ucsd.edu/

22 https://www.colorado.gov/pacific/cdphe/medical-marijuana-research-grants

23 http://learnaboutmarijuanawa.org/research.htm

24 Chris Duvall, Cannabis, Reaktion Books, 2015, pg. 15

25 Duvall, ibid

26 Isaac Campos, Home Grown - Marijuana and the Origins of Mexico's War on Drugs, The University of North Carolina Press, 2012

27 John C. McWilliams, The Protectors - Harry J. Anslinger and the Federal Bureau of Narcotics, 1930-1962. Associated University Presses. 1990.

28 American Civil Liberties Union, "The War on Marijuana in Black and White." https://www.aclu.org/report/war-marijuana-black-and-white

29 ThirdWay.org poll; 2014; http://www.thirdway.org/report/the-marijuana-middle-americans-ponder-legalization;

30 Harris Poll, 2015, http://www.theharrispoll.com/politics/Americans-Ready-for-Legal-Marijuana.html

31 http://lawyers.norml.org/

32 Guzman, IACM, http://www.cannabis-med.org/index.php?tpl=faq&red=faqlist&id=274&lng=en

33 2009, Oxford University Press.

34 http://www.ncsl.org/research/health/state-medical-marijuana-laws.aspx

35 http://www.cancer.gov/about-cancer/treatment/cam/hp/cannabis-pdq

36 http://www.projectcbd.org/about-project-cbd

37 https://www.clinicaltrials.gov/ct2/results?term=marijuana&recr=Open

38 http://cannabis-med.org/data/pdf/2001-03-04-7.pdf

39 Taming THC: potential cannabis synergy and phytocannabinoid-terpenoid entourage effects Ethan B Russo, GW Pharmaceuticals, British Journal of Pharmacology, Cannabinoids in Biology and Medicine, Part I, 2011, DOI:10.1111/j.1476-5381.2011.01238.x

40 Cannabis and Cannabis Extracts: Greater Than the Sum of Their Parts? John M. McPartland, Ethan B. Russo, Journal of Cannabis Ther- apeutics (The Haworth Integrative Healing Press, an imprint of The Haworth Press, Inc.) Vol. 1, No. 3/4, 2001, pp. 103-132; and: Cannabis Therapeutics in HIV/AIDS (ed: Ethan Russo) The Haworth Integrative Healing Press, an imprint of The Haworth Press, Inc., 2001, pp. 103-132.

41 http://onlinelibrary.wiley.com/store/10.111

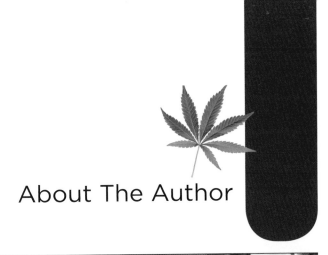

About The Author

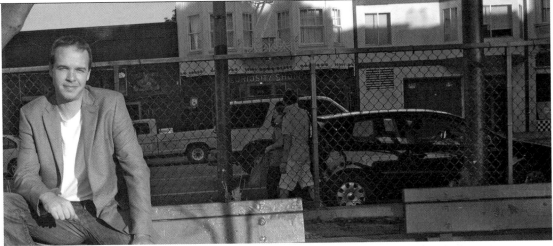

David Downs is an award-winning freelance journalist, and best-selling author whose work has appeared in *The New York Times*, *WIRED*, *Rolling Stone*, *The Onion*, *San Francisco Chronicle*, *Billboard Magazine*, and many other fine publications.

Downs is the author, co-author, or contributing writer of two other cannabis-related books: the best-seller *Beyond Buds* (2014), and *Marijuana Harvest* (2016).

Downs covers cannabis policy and legalization in the award-winning syndicated column "Legalization Nation," published by the *East Bay Express* newspaper in Oakland, California. Downs reports and edits the cannabis culture blog "Smell the Truth" on SFGate.com — a leading Internet news source. Downs also reviews cannabis products and covers national stories as a contributing writer for *CULTURE* magazine. Downs also co-founded leading cannabis podcast, *The Hash*, found at TheHash.org, and co-founded the cannabis technology, finance and media summit — the New West Summit.

He holds a bachelor's degree in English Literature from UC Santa Barbara, and was a Fellow at the Medill School of Journalism's Academy of Alternative Journalism in Chicago. Downs is a guest lecturer at UC Berkeley, and a contributor to Continuing Education of the Bar's Marijuana Law Hub, sponsored by University of California and the State Bar of California.

The author lives in San Francisco with his wife and two children.

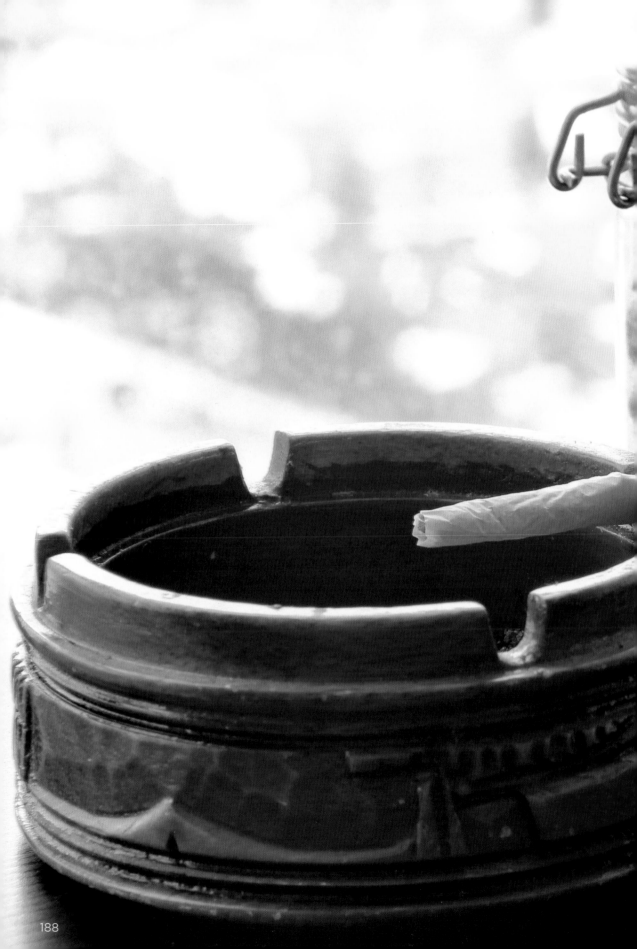

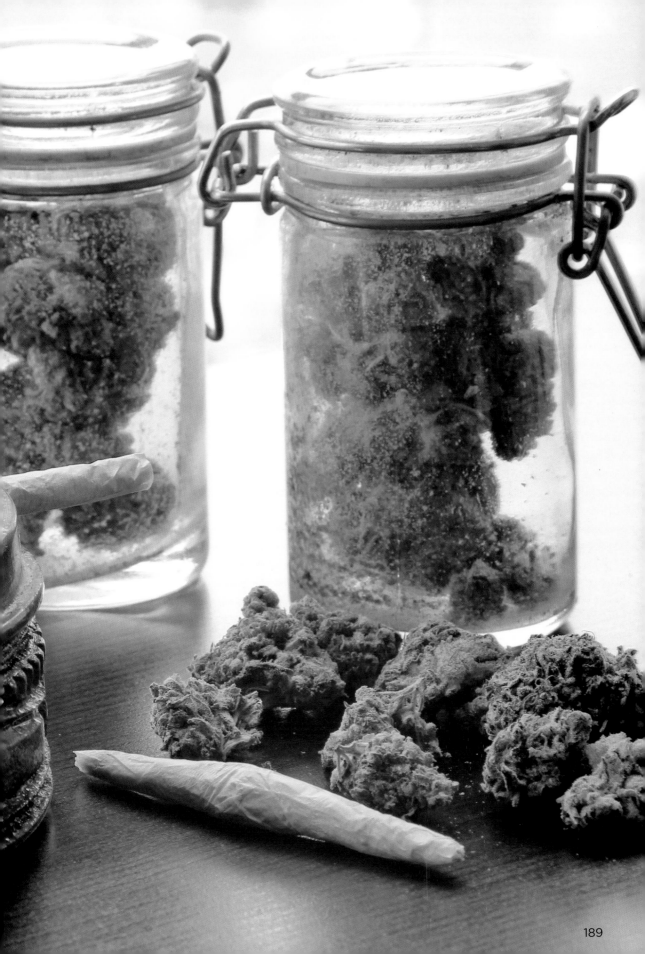

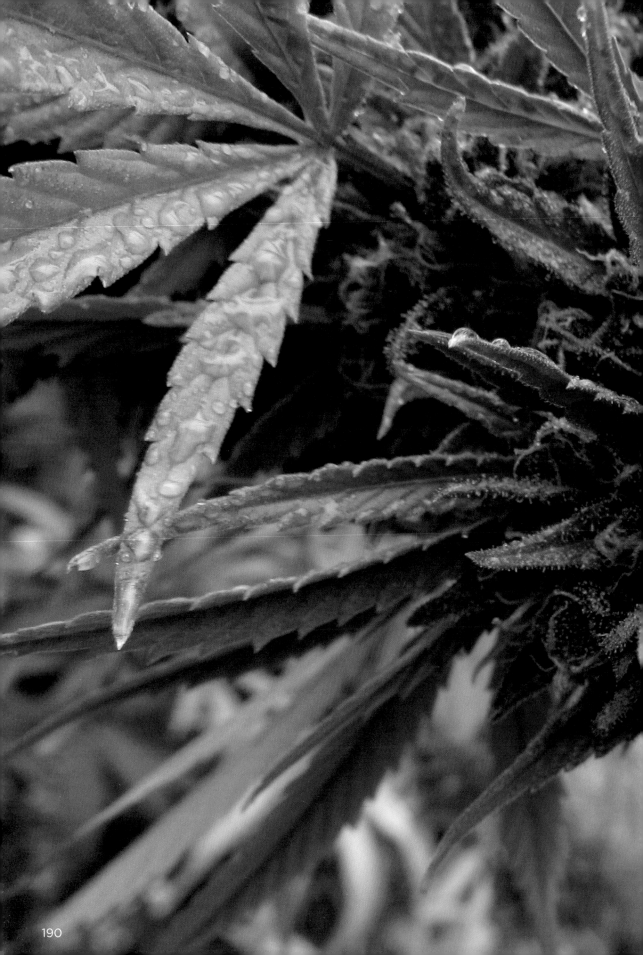

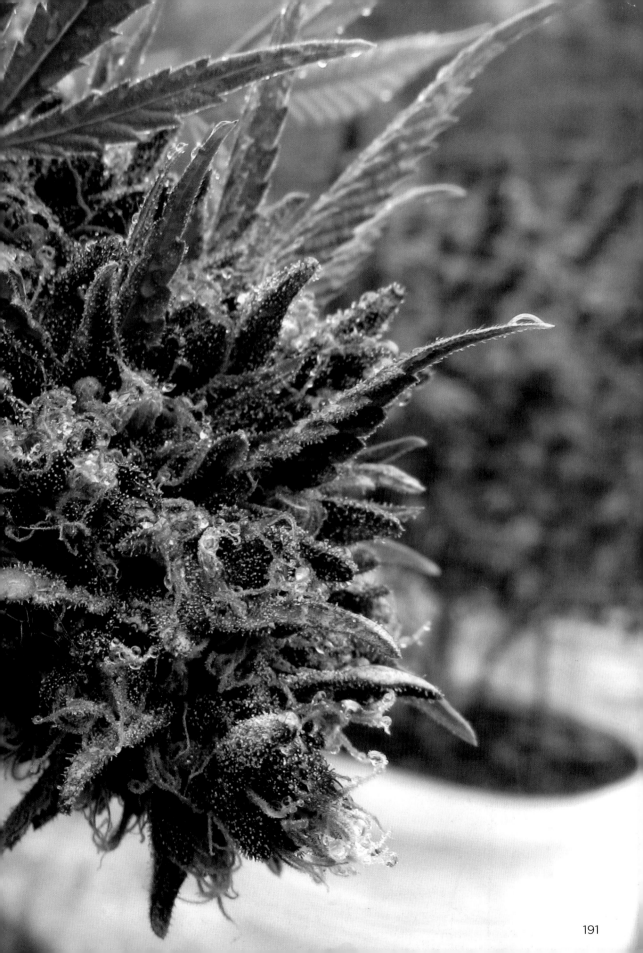

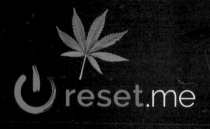